T0383373

Respiratory Viruses in Pediatric and Adult Populations

Guest Editor

ALEXANDER J. McADAM, MD, PhD

CLINICS IN LABORATORY MEDICINE

www.labmed.theclinics.com

Consulting Editor
ALAN WELLS, MD, DMSc

December 2009 • Volume 29 • Number 4

SAUNDERS an imprint of ELSEVIER, Inc.

W.B. SAUNDERS COMPANY
A Division of Elsevier Inc.

1600 John F. Kennedy Boulevard • Suite 1800 • Philadelphia, Pennsylvania 19103-2899

http://www.theclinics.com

CLINICS IN LABORATORY MEDICINE Volume 29, Number 4

December 2009 ISSN 0272-2712, ISBN-13: 978-1-4377-1517-0, ISBN-10: 1-4377-1517-6

Editor: Katie Hartner
Developmental Editor: Donald Mumford

Reprints. For copies of 100 or more, of articles in this publication, please contact the Commercial Reprints Department, Elsevier Inc., 360 Park Avenue South, New York, New York 10010-1710. Tel. (212) 633-3813, Fax: (212) 462-1935, E-mail: reprints@elsevier.com.

Clinics in Laboratory Medicine (ISSN 0272-2712) is published quarterly by Elsevier Inc., 360 Park Avenue South, New York, NY 10010-1710. Months of issue are March, June, September, and December. Business and Editorial offices: 1600 John F. Kennedy Blvd., Suite 1800, Philadelphia, PA 19103-2899. Periodicals postage paid at New York, NY and additional mailing offices. Subscription prices are $220.00 per year (US individuals), $347.00 per year (US institutions), $114.00 (US students), $253.00 per year (Canadian individuals), $438.00 per year (foreign institutions), $157.00 (foreign students). Foreign air speed delivery is included in all *Clinics* subscription prices. All prices are subject to change without notice. POSTMASTER: Send address changes to *Clinics in Laboratory Medicine*, Elsevier Health Sciences Division, Subscription Customer Service, 3251 Riverport Lane, Maryland Heights, MO 63043. **Customer Service: 1-800-654-2452 (US). From outside of the US and Canada, call 1-314-447-8871. Fax: 1-314-447-8029. E-mail: journalscustomerservice-usa@elsevier.com (for print support) or journalsonlinesupport-usa@elsevier.com (for online support).**

Clinics in Laboratory Medicine is covered in *EMBASE/Exerpta Medica, MEDLINE/PubMed (Index Medicus), Cinahl, Current Contents/Clinical Medicine, BIOSIS* and *ISI/BIOMED.*

Printed and bound by CPI Group (UK) Ltd, Croydon, CR0 4YY

Transferred to Digital Print 2011

Contributors

GUEST EDITOR

ALEXANDER J. McADAM, MD, PhD
Department of Laboratory Medicine, Children's Hospital Boston, Boston, Massachusetts

AUTHORS

CARLOS A. CAMARGO, Jr, MD, DrPH
Associate Professor of Medicine, Department of Emergency Medicine, Division of Rheumatology, Allergy, and Immunology, Department of Medicine, Massachusetts General Hospital, Harvard Medical School, Boston, Massachusetts

BRIAN D.W. CHOW, MD
Case Western Reserve University, Cleveland, Ohio; Department of Pediatrics, University Hospitals Case Medical Center, Cleveland, Ohio; Department of Internal Medicine, University Hospitals Case Medical Center, Cleveland, Ohio

FRANK P. ESPER, MD
Case Western Reserve University, Cleveland, Ohio; Department of Pediatrics, University Hospitals Case Medical Center, Cleveland, Ohio; Division of Pediatric Infectious Diseases, Rainbow Babies and Children's Hospital, Cleveland, Ohio

SUSANNA ESPOSITO, MD
Associate Professor of Pediatrics, Department of Maternal and Pediatric Sciences, University of Milan, Fondazione IRCCS Ospedale Maggiore Policlinico, Mangiagalli e Regina Elena, Via Commenda, Milano, Italy

SUE C. KEHL, PhD
Associate Professor, Department of Pathology, Medical College of Wisconsin, Milwaukee, WI; Associate Director, Clinical Pathology and Technical Director, Microbiology, Children's Hospital of Wisconsin, Milwaukee, WI

SWATI KUMAR, MD
Assistant Professor of Pediatrics, Division of Infectious Diseases, Medical College of Wisconsin, Milwaukee, WI; Infectious Diseases Physician, Children's Hospital of Wisconsin, Milwaukee, WI

MARIE LOUISE LANDRY, MD
Professor, Department of Laboratory Medicine, Yale University School of Medicine, New Haven, Connecticut; Clinical Virology Laboratory, Yale New Haven Hospital, New Haven, Connecticut

JONATHAN M. MANSBACH, MD
Assistant Professor of Pediatrics, Department of Medicine, Children's Hospital Boston, Harvard Medical School, Boston, Massachusetts

ALEXANDER J. McADAM, MD, PhD
Associate Professor of Pathology, Department of Pathology, Harvard Medical School, Massachusetts; Medical Director Infectious Diseases Diagnostic Division, Department of Laboratory Medicine, Children's Hospital Boston, Boston, Massachusetts

YOSHIHIKO MURATA, MD, PhD
Assistant Professor of Medicine, Division of Infectious Diseases, Department of Medicine, University of Rochester School of Medicine and Dentistry, Rochester, New York; Attending Physician, Infectious Diseases Unit, Rochester General Hospital, Rochester, New York

NICOLA PRINCIPI, MD
Professor of Pediatrics, Department of Maternal and Pediatric Sciences, University of Milan, Fondazione IRCCS Ospedale Maggiore Policlinico, Mangiagalli e Regina Elena, Via Commenda, Milano, Italy

ANN MARIE RILEY, BS
Virology Supervisor, Infectious Diseases Diagnostic Division, Department of Laboratory Medicine, Children's Hospital Boston, Boston, Massachusetts

YI-WEI TANG, MD, PhD
Department of Pathology, Vanderbilt University Medical Center, Nashville, Tennessee; Department of Medicine, Vanderbilt University Medical Center, Nashville, Tennessee; Molecular Infectious Disease Laboratory, Vanderbilt University Hospital, Nashville, Tennessee

LIA VAN DER HOEK, PhD
Laboratory of Experimental Virology, Department of Medical Microbiology Center for Infection and Immunity (CINIMA), Academic Medical Center (AMC), Amsterdam, The Netherlands

BRIGITTE A. WEVERS, MSc
Master Biomedical Sciences, VU University Amsterdam, Faculty of Earth and Life Sciences, Amsterdam, The Netherlands

WENJUAN WU, PhD
Department of Pathology, Vanderbilt University Medical Center, Nashville, Tennessee; Shanghai Public Health Clinical Center, Fudan University, Shanghai, People's Republic of China

Contents

Viral culture is the historical gold standard for detection of most viruses that cause respiratory tract infections. Viral culture remains valuable because it is reasonably sensitive for most respiratory viruses, and it is cheaper and less technically demanding than nucleic acid amplified tests. The disadvantages of conventional viral culture using multiple tubes of cell lines are that it is labor intensive, moderately expensive, and slow. Advances in viral culture include the introduction of new cell lines, which can be more sensitive or convenient than previously used cell lines, and the use of shell-vial culture for respiratory viruses. Shell-vial culture is as sensitive as conventional culture for most respiratory viruses and it has a much shorter turn-around time. The shorter turn-around time increases the clinical utility of these cultures.

In most hospitals, clinics, and doctor's offices, immunologic assays are the only tests performed on site for the diagnosis of respiratory viruses. More than other methods, immunoassays have been shown to affect patient management and save costs, aiding early administration of antiviral therapy, reduction in unnecessary tests and antibiotics, and earlier discharges. This article discusses the major immunologic methods employed for respiratory virus diagnosis, recent developments in immunoassays and sample collection, and current test algorithms.

This article describes the clinical and socioeconomic relevance of influenza (IV) and respiratory syncytial virus (RSV) in pediatrics, the characteristics and limitations of currently available assays, and the impact of rapid diagnostic tests. This article shows that rapid tests for the detection and identification of IV and RSV in the respiratory secretions of infants and children are useful in the diagnosis of common, and possibly severe diseases, such as influenza and bronchiolitis. The tests' specificity and sensitivity make them most reliable when the prevalence of influenza or RSV infection is high, which suggests that their routine use should be restricted to the peak periods of viral circulation. The most recently marketed tests are similarly effective in identifying viruses, and so pediatricians should choose those that are less expensive, less time consuming, and easier to perform and to interpret.

Viruses are major contributors to morbidity and mortality from acute respiratory infections in all age groups worldwide. Accurate identification of the etiologic agent of respiratory tract infections is important for proper patient management. Diagnosis can be problematic, because a range of potential pathogens can cause similar clinical symptoms. Nucleic acid amplification testing is emerging as the preferred method of diagnostic testing. Real-time technology and the ability to perform multiplex testing have facilitated this emergence. Commercial platforms for nucleic acid amplification testing of respiratory viruses include real-time polymerase chain reaction (PCR), nucleic acid sequence-based amplification, and loop-mediated isothermal amplification. Multiplex PCR with fluidic microarrays or DNA chips are the most recent diagnostic advance. These assays offer significant advantages in sensitivity over antigen detection methods and in most cases also over traditional culture methods. A limited number of assays, however, are commercially available, thus laboratory developed assays frequently are used. This article reviews the performance of commercially available assays and discusses issues relevant to the development of in-house assays.

This article describes several emerging molecular assays that have potential applications in the diagnosis and monitoring of respiratory viral infections. These techniques include direct nucleic acid detection by quantum dots, loop-mediated isothermal amplification, multiplex ligation-dependent probe amplification, amplification using arbitrary primers, target-enriched multiplexing amplification, pyrosequencing, padlock probes, solid and suspension microarrays, and mass spectrometry. Several of these systems already are commercially available to provide multiplex amplification and high-throughput detection and identification of a panel of respiratory viral pathogens. Further validation and implementation of such emerging molecular assays in routine clinical virology services will enhance the rapid diagnosis of respiratory viral infections and improve patient care.

Respiratory tract infections are a leading cause of morbidity and mortality worldwide. The human bocavirus (HBoV) is a newly recognized human

children who have severe bronchiolitis (eg, an episode requiring hospitalization) will develop recurrent wheezing or asthma. Although many environmental and genetic factors may play a role in the pathway from bronchiolitis to asthma, this article focuses on the viruses that have been linked to bronchiolitis and how these viruses may predict or contribute to future wheezing and asthma. The article also discusses vitamin D as an emerging risk factor for respiratory infections and wheezing.

THE CLINICS ARE NOW AVAILABLE ONLINE!

Access your subscription at:
www.theclinics.com

Preface

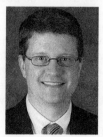

Alexander J. McAdam, MD, PhD
Guest Editor

Respiratory viruses continue to be a fascinating subject. The mutability of these viruses leads to the periodic emergence of new serotypes or species of viruses as human pathogens. Because these viruses are readily transmitted, a new respiratory virus that emerges can spread rapidly. The coronavirus associated with the severe acute respiratory syndrome (SARS) and the novel influenza A (H1N1) virus (swine influenza) are two examples of respiratory viruses that spread very quickly after emerging. According to data from the World Health Organization, there have been 55,867 cases and 238 deaths due to the H1N1 virus to date (http://www.who.int/csr/don/2009_06_24/en/index.html, accessed June 25, 2009). This outbreak underscores the importance of our continued attention to the epidemiology, manifestations, and diagnosis of respiratory viruses.

Viral culture and immunological assays have been the mainstays of viral diagnosis for decades. These methods are cheaper and technically simpler than the currently available molecular methods, but they are less sensitive than nucleic acid amplified tests (NAATs). Recent improvements in viral culture and immunoassays have led to increased sensitivity, reduced turnaround time, and the ability to detect recently discovered viruses. These improvements are described in the articles by Ms. Riley and myself who discuss viral culture, and Dr. Landry, who discusses immunological assays. Drs. Principi and Esposito extend the discussion of immunoassays with an article on the utility of rapid immunoassays for influenza virus and respiratory syncytial virus (RSV) in children.

There is a revolution underway in the methods for diagnosis of respiratory viruses. NAATs have greatly improved the sensitivity of detection of these viruses. Sophisticated laboratories have been performing user-designed ("home brew") assays or analyte-specific reagent-based tests, but the recent introduction of NAATs approved by the Food and Drug Administration (FDA) for respiratory viruses will begin to make NAATs accessible to more laboratories. FDA-approved NAATs are discussed by Drs. Kehl and Kumar, who also discuss some important issues to consider in the design of user-developed assays. We take a look at the exciting future of molecular methods of testing for respiratory viruses in the article by Drs. Wu and Tang.

Clin Lab Med 29 (2009) xi–xii
doi:10.1016/j.cll.2009.07.012
0272-2712/09/$ – see front matter © 2009 Elsevier Inc. All rights reserved.

labmed.theclinics.com

New respiratory viruses continue be discovered. Cutting-edge methods have led to the discovery of several viruses that have presumably infected humans for decades, but which have only recently come to our attention. The recently discovered bocaviruses and the current controversy about the role of these viruses in disease are discussed in the article by Drs. Chow and Esper. Two strains of coronaviruses that were recently discovered (HCoV-NL63 and HCoV-HKU1), but which have presumably infected humans for a long time, are discussed by Drs. Wevers and van der Hoek. These authors also discuss a truly new human pathogen, the SARS coronavirus, which caused the highly lethal outbreak of SARS in 2002 to 2003. These newly discovered viruses remind us that there is still a great deal to be learned about respiratory virus infections, and that continued research is needed.

Recent developments in clinical aspects of respiratory virus infections are discussed in the final two articles in this volume. Dr Murata discusses the problematic history of development of a vaccine for RSV and, more importantly, the several avenues of current investigation that might lead to a vaccine for RSV. The role of respiratory viruses in bronchiolitis and in asthma is discussed by Drs Mansbach and Camargo. These authors also review some very recent and interesting data that suggest that levels of vitamin D may be related to wheezing and asthma.

I enjoyed reading these reviews and I hope you do, too. They represent the most current information about respiratory viruses by leaders in the field. This area of laboratory medicine is advancing quickly, with new diagnostic tests and viruses appearing frequently, and for that reason it continues to be very exciting.

Alexander J. McAdam, MD, PhD
Department of Laboratory Medicine
Children's Hospital Boston
300 Longwood Avenue
Boston, MA 02115, USA

E-mail address:
Alexander.McAdam@childrens.harvard.edu

Developments in Tissue Culture Detection of Respiratory Viruses

Alexander J. McAdam, MD, PhD[a,b,]*, Ann Marie Riley, BS[b]

KEYWORDS

- Viral culture • Shell vial viral culture • Influenza virus
- Respiratory syncytial virus • Parainfluenza virus • Adenovirus

There are now several technologies available for detection of viruses, including those viruses which frequently cause respiratory tract infections. The available methods range from insensitive, but technically simple and inexpensive, point-of-care tests to highly sensitive, but technically challenging and expensive, nucleic acid amplification tests (NAAT). While viral culture is moderately technically challenging, it is simpler than NAAT and it has advantages over immunoassays in sensitivity for some viruses and for the types of viruses that can be readily detected.

The focus of this article is on improvements in the utility of viral culture for detection of respiratory viruses. Detection of viruses from clinical specimens is the main subject, but the use of viral culture for testing the susceptibility of influenza A and B viruses to some anti-viral drugs is also discussed. Viral culture is also a method for production of viruses, and has current and potential applications in research and vaccine development; however, it is beyond the scope of this article.

PROBLEMS WITH CONVENTIONAL VIRAL CULTURE FOR RESPIRATORY VIRUSES

For this article, we consider conventional viral culture for respiratory viruses to mean culture of respiratory samples in tubes of several types of mammalian cells that are chosen to support detection of influenza viruses, respiratory syncytial viruses (RSV), parainfluenza viruses, adenoviruses, and sometimes, rhinoviruses.[1] Typically, three or four cell types are inoculated with the specimen (sometimes in duplicate) and these cultures are incubated for 10 to 14 days, or longer in a few laboratories. Each tube is periodically checked for the presence of replicating virus by hemadsorption (HA) for

[a] Department of Pathology, Harvard Medical School, 77 Avenue Louis Pasteur, Boston, MA 02115, USA
[b] Infectious Diseases Diagnostic Division, Department of Laboratory Medicine, Children's Hospital Boston, 300 Longwood Avenue, Boston, MA 02115, USA
* Corresponding author. Infectious Diseases Diagnostic Division, Department of Laboratory Medicine, Children's Hospital Boston, 300 Longwood Avenue, Boston, MA 02115.
E-mail address: Alexander.McAdam@childrens.harvard.edu (A. McAdam).

Clin Lab Med 29 (2009) 623–634
doi:10.1016/j.cll.2009.07.009
0272-2712/09/$ – see front matter © 2009 Elsevier Inc. All rights reserved.

labmed.theclinics.com

influenza and parainfluenza viruses, and by microscopy for cytopathic effect (CPE) for the other viruses. Once HA or CPE has been detected, the presence of the suspected viruses is confirmed by staining the cells by immunofluorescence.

This simple description of conventional viral culture makes the problems with this method clear: it is slow, it is a lot of work, and the supplies are expensive. The length of time it takes to detect viruses by conventional viral culture reduces the clinical utility of the result. Reporting the presence of influenza virus in a day will have more clinical impact than reporting it in a week.

Why perform viral culture on respiratory specimens at all? Even the fastest methods of viral culture take one or two days, while immunoassays can be performed in 1 hour or less. NAAT are more sensitive than viral culture and can be performed in a few days or less, depending on the workflow. All of these tests have reasonable specificity when they are correctly performed. Nevertheless, the modern methods of viral culture for respiratory viruses described in this article will continue to be a good choice for many laboratories. The advantages of viral culture are first, that it is more sensitive than immunoassays for most respiratory viruses, and second, that it is far simpler and cheaper than NAAT. Until NAAT become easier to perform, probably through automation, and less expensive, viral culture for respiratory viruses will continue to be useful.

In the rest of this article, we discuss newly described cell lines that can be used for viral culture and the use of shell-vial culture for detection of respiratory viruses.

NEWLY DESCRIBED CELL LINES FOR CULTURE OF RESPIRATORY VIRUSES
Genetically Modified Madin-Darby Canine Kidney Cells

Madin-Darby canine kidney (MDCK) cells are an established cell line that can be used to grow and detect influenza viruses.[1] They are a convenient alternative to primary monkey kidney (PMK) cells for influenza virus culture. MDCK cells have been genetically modified to express higher levels of the molecule bound by the viral hemagglutinin and neuraminidase proteins present on the surface of influenza virus strains adapted to growth in human hosts. Influenza viruses bind to host cells through the binding of viral hemagglutinin protein to sialyloligosaccharides on the host-cell surface.[2] After replication, exit of influenza virus from the host cell depends on cleavage of sialic acid from the saccharides on the host cell. The structure of the sialyloligosaccharides differs between different animal species, and the influenza viruses that grow in a given host species preferentially bind and cleave the specific sialyloligosaccharides found in that species. Most of the terminal N-acetyl sialic acid residues on human respiratory epithelial cells are bound to the saccharide in an $\alpha2,6$-linkage (called NeuAc$\alpha2,6$Gal), and so influenza viruses from humans would be expected to replicate well in cells with surface NeuAc$\alpha2,6$Gal.[2] While MDCK cells do have NeuAc$\alpha2,6$Gal on their surface, they also have a second type of cell-surface sialic acid (NeuAc$\alpha2,3$Gal).[3] By increasing the level of NeuAc$\alpha2,6$Gal and decreasing the level of NeuAc$\alpha2,3$Gal present on the surface of MDCK cells, one might be able to make MDCK cells better able to support replication of influenza viruses from human infections.

MDCK cells have been genetically modified to express the gene for an enzyme that catalyzes the α-2,6-sialylation of N-acetyllactosamine (the SIAT1 gene).[3] Compared with control MDCK cells, the MDCK-SIAT1 cells have approximately twofold higher levels of NeuAc$\alpha2,6$Gal and twofold lower levels of NeuAc$\alpha2,3$Gal.[3] As expected, an influenza A (H1N1) strain adapted to growth in humans binds with greater affinity to the MDCK-SIAT1 cells than to control MDCK cells. When the same strain of influenza A virus was adapted to growth in embryonated chicken eggs, it did not have the preferential affinity for the MDCK-SIAT1 cells. These data suggest that increased expression of NeuAcα2,6Gal would make the MDCK-SIAT1 cells better able to support replication of influenza viruses from human infections.

MDCK-SIAT1 cells were created for use in a functional assay for resistance of influenza virus to neuraminidase inhibitors (eg, oseltamivir, brand name Tamiflu).[3] Neuraminidase inhibitors are used to reduce the illness caused by influenza virus infection, but resistance can develop during treatment. During the winters of 2007 to 2008 and 2008 to 2009 many isolates of influenza A (H1N1) were resistant to oseltamivir.[4] Cell lines used for influenza virus culture, including MDCK cells, do not give accurate results in functional assays for oseltamivir resistance, probably because expression of low levels of NeuAcα2,6Gal lead to apparent oseltamivir insensitivity even when the virus is susceptible to the drug.[3] Unlike MDCK cells, MDCK-SIAT1 cells allow ready detection of oseltamivir resistance in a bioassay.[3] Matrosovich and colleagues used two wild-type oseltamivir susceptible influenza A strains and their corresponding oseltamivir resistant mutants in a bioassay with MDCK-SIAT1 cells and found that the resistant mutants demonstrated 100-fold, or greater, resistance to oseltamivir.[3] Hatakeyama and colleagues tested a larger number of influenza virus isolates (six H3N2, six H1N1 and five influenza B) in a bioassay for oseltamivir susceptibility with independently generated MDCK engineered to express increased levels of NeuAcα2,6Gal (which they called ST6Gal I cells).[5] They found that reduction of plaque size by 50% in greater than 90% of plaques, rather than plaque number, accurately reflected the susceptibility of the viruses to oseltamivir. The gold standard for oseltamivir susceptibility in this study was an in vitro assay for the concentration of oseltamivir which inhibited 50% of the sialidase activity of neuraminidase. Taken together, these studies demonstrate that MDCK-SIAT1 is a good bioassay for oseltamivir susceptibility in influenza A and B viruses.

There are intriguing data which indicate that MDCK-SIAT1 cells could be used in a sensitive cell culture assay for influenza viruses. Hatakeyama and colleagues compared ST6Gal I cells with control MDCK cells for detection of influenza virus in 20 clinical specimens known to contain influenza viruses.[5] The clinical specimens were titrated with the control MDCK cells and ST6Gal I cells, cultured with media containing trypsin (to enhance plaque formation), and then stained for viral plaques after 2 or 3 days. Eight specimens had influenza A (H3N2), seven had influenza A (H1N1), and five had influenza B. Influenza virus was detected in all 20 specimens using the ST6Gal I cells, but in only 10 of 20 specimens using the MDCK cells (three influenza A (H3N2), six influenza A (H1N1), and one influenza B). Furthermore, the replication efficiency of influenza viruses previously grown in MDCK cells was greater in ST6Gal I cells than in MDCK cells, and plaques formed in the transfectants were larger and easier to visualize.

In a separate study, Oh and colleagues used MDCK-SIAT1 cells and MDCK for detection of influenza virus from a large number (125) of specimens known to contain influenza virus (39 influenza A (H1N1), 53 influenza A (H3N2), and 33 influenza B).[6] After 4 days of growth, the supernatant was tested for influenza virus by hemagglutination. Two thirds of the isolates were detected from cell lines, one third were detected only from the MDCK-SIAT1 cells, and none were detected only from the MDCK cells. The titer of virus obtained from clinical specimens was higher in the MDCK-SIAT1 cells than in MDCK cells for influenza A isolates, but the two cell lines yielded similar titers of influenza B. The repeated passage of influenza viruses in MDCK and MDCK-SIAT1 cells does lead to mutations in the genes encoding the viral hemagglutinin protein, but the frequency of mutation was the same regardless of which cell was used.[6]

To date, there are no studies that we are aware of that determine whether MDCK cells modified to express high levels of NeuAcα2,6Gal are superior to unmodified

MDCK cells, or to primary monkey kidney cells, when used for routine methods of detection of influenza virus from clinical specimens. The studies discussed earlier use small numbers of samples or methods of viral detection that are unlikely to be used in routine diagnostic laboratories (eg, plaque assays). However, these studies do demonstrate that most influenza A and B isolates that have been tested grow to higher titer in the engineered MDCK cells than in control MDCK cells, and they provide promising, if limited, data suggesting that these cells could be routinely used in a sensitive influenza virus assay.

HuH7 Cells

HuH7 cells are human hepatocellular carcinoma cells. These cells, and other human hepatocellular carcinoma cell lines, have the interesting feature that they produce little or no type I interferons (IFN-α and IFN-β) in response to viral infection.[7] Interferons are cytokines that are produced in response to viral infection and that cause neighboring cells to reduce permissiveness for viral replication. In addition to producing little or no type I interferons, HuH7 cells show reduced viral replication only with very high levels of type I interferons.[7] These findings suggest that HuH7 cells might support viral replication well, and could be useful in detection of viruses by viral culture.

Freymuth and colleagues have described the use of HuH7 cells for viral culture with respiratory viruses.[8,9] They cultured HuH7 cells in 24 well plates to 80% confluence, and inoculated the cells with specimen by centrifugation, as would be done with shell-vial cultures. The cells were examined for CPE for 4 days and then analyzed by either direct fluorescence assay (DFA) or by NAAT on the culture supernatant. They tested the ability of HuH7 cells to support replication of culture-adapted isolates of influenza A, influenza B, RSV, human metapneumovirus, coronaviruses, parainfluenza viruses types 1, 2, 3, and 4, adenoviruses, enteroviruses and rhinoviruses. CPE was detectable with all tested isolates of influenza viruses, parainfluenza viruses, coronavirus, rhinovirus and most (19 of 21) adenovirus. There was no detectable CPE with RSV or human metapneumovirus, although replication of these viruses could be detected by immunofluorescence or reverse transcription polymerase chain reaction, respectively. Although the rate of replication of influenza viruses in HuH7 cells was slower than in MDCK cells, all isolates of influenza viruses could be detected with the HuH7 cells.

These authors also described the use of HuH7 cells as part of routine viral culture.[8] They used HuH7 cells for viral culture of specimens that were negative by immunofluorescence for influenza A and B viruses, RSV, parainfluenza viruses 1, 2, and 3, and adenovirus. Viral culture with HuH7 cells detected a large number of influenza A and B viruses that were missed by immunofluorescence (approximately 30% more of each detected), and parainfluenza 1 (31.7%), parainfluenza 2 (55.5%) and adenovirus (21.1%). A smaller yield was found with HuH7 viral culture for detecting RSV (1.2% more detected than IF) and parainfluenza 3 (11.4%), but given that immunofluorescence is sensitive for these two viruses, this is not surprising. Several viruses that were not tested for immunofluorescence, but that were detected by HuH7 viral culture, included rhinovirus, enterovirus, and coronavirus. HuH7 cells also support replication of coronaviruses, including the severe acute respiratory syndrome (SARS) coronavirus.[9,10]

HuH7 cells appear to be a good alternative to other cell lines for detection of influenza viruses, parainfluenza viruses, and adenoviruses, and also allow detection of at least some isolates of rhinovirus, enterovirus, and coronavirus. Unfortunately, there are no comprehensive comparisons of the sensitivity of HuH7 cells to alternative cell lines, such as MDCK or A549 cells for detection of all of these viruses. Such a comparison would be very useful in determining how these cells would be best used in the diagnostic virology laboratory.

SHELL-VIAL CULTURE FOR RESPIRATORY VIRUSES

Shell-vial viral culture has the advantage of giving faster results than conventional (tube) viral culture. Shell-vial culture is performed by centrifuging the specimen onto a monolayer of cells on a coverslip in the bottom of a vial.[1] The culture is incubated for 1 to 4 days before being stained for the presence of virus by immunofluorescence. There is little, if anything, to be gained by reading shell-vial cultures for CPE and this is usually not done. The centrifugation is long (eg, 30 to 60 minutes) and slow (eg, 700 x gravity), and this enhances the viral infectivity.[1] The mechanism by which shell-vial culture increases sensitivity is not known. The selection of which cell types are used, the days that the shell vials are stained, and of course, the specificity of the antibodies used, all determine what viruses can be detected.

As previously mentioned, the main advantage of shell-vial culture is that viruses are detected more quickly than by conventional culture. There is little need for longer incubation times because most viruses are detected within 1 or 2 days. Another advantage of shell-vial cultures is a reduction in labor compared with conventional viral culture, which can reduce the cost of the test. There are two potential disadvantages to shell-vial culture. First, if the method is not optimized, shell-vial culture can be less sensitive than conventional culture, and this insensitivity must be carefully assessed before shell-vial culture is adopted. Second, shell-vial culture will only detect the viruses that are supported by the cell lines used and that are detected by the antibody used. As a result, shell-vial cultures typically detect fewer types of virus than a conventional viral culture. But progress has been made in increasing the number of viruses that a shell vial can detect by using multiple cell types in a single vial, and by staining the monolayer with multiple antibodies.

We briefly review the use of shell-vial culture to detect a single type of respiratory virus, but these methods have become less useful as methods for the detection of multiple respiratory viruses in a single shell vial have become common. The latter is the focus of this section, as this is the method of viral culture likely to be adopted by most laboratories which consider shell-vial culture for respiratory viruses.

Shell-Vial Cultures for Single Respiratory Viruses

Most studies of the use of shell-vial culture for influenza A and B viruses have used PMK cells, as these are the preferred cells for conventional culture of influenza viruses. The sensitivity of shell vial for influenza viruses is lower than conventional culture with PMK cells. In one study, conventional culture detected influenza A or B in 82 samples; only 30 of these were detected by shell vial, and shell vial detected another 12 that were negative in conventional culture.[11] Conventional culture took 3.6 and 4.3 days to detect influenza A and B, respectively, while shell vials were completed at 2 days.[11] Another study using PMK cells found that all specimens positive for influenza A or B were detected by conventional culture, although only 60% of these were detected by shell-vial culture.[12] Cell lines that can be grown for diagnostic use are more convenient for viral culture than primary cells. One study compared three cell lines for use in shell-vial culture detection of influenza virus.[13] MDCK cells were 100% sensitive, which was significantly higher than the sensitivity of Vero cells (71.4%) or MRC-5 cells (57.1%). PMK cells were not included in this study, either in shell-vial or conventional-viral culture, so the relative sensitivities of PMK and MDCK cells in shell-vial testing was not determined.

HEp-2 cells can be used for shell-vial culture of RSV. The sensitivity of shell-vial culture for RSV is equal to, or higher, than conventional culture. Sensitivities of shell-vial cultures for RSV range from 73% to 92%, while the sensitivities of conventional cultures in the same studies range from 58.4% to 90%.[14–17] Out of 46 specimens that were positive for RSV by shell vial in one study, 43 (93.5%) were detected on the first day, 3 (6.5%) more were detected on the second day, and no additional positives were detected on the third day.[16] In the same study, it took 2 to 8 days to detect RSV by conventional culture, with an average of 4.5 days. Immunofluorescence is typically more sensitive than culture for RSV, but if culture for RSV is done, shell-vial culture can be recommended as being as sensitive, or slightly more sensitive, compared with conventional culture, but with shorter turn-around time.

Shell-Vial Cultures for Multiple Respiratory Viruses

Several shell-vial viral culture systems have been tested for the detection of panels of respiratory viruses. Typically, these are designed to detect influenza A and B viruses, RSV, adenovirus, and parainfluenza viruses (types 1, 2, and 3). To be adequately sensitive for each of these viruses, two cell lines are used. Most cell types will support proliferation of each of the viruses to differing degrees, but in general the shell-vial cultures include a cell line that supports replication of RSV and adenovirus (eg, HEp-2, A549) and another cell line to support replication of influenza, parainfluenza, and adenovirus (eg, PMK, MDCK). Separate shell vials are usually used for each cell type, but one commercial product combines multiple cell lines in a single shell vial (see later discussion). The number of shell vials of each type inoculated will depend on the number of time points on which vials are harvested for staining by immunofluorescence (usually one or two time points), and the staining strategy, as discussed next.

Immunofluorescence for detection of multiple viruses can be done in two general ways. First, the cells can be scraped off the cover slip, spotted in multiple wells of a slide, and then dried and fixed. Next, one well can be stained by immunofluorescence for each of the viruses separately, for a total of approximately seven stains. Alternatively, the cells can be stained for immunofluorescence using a pool of antibodies against all the viruses to be detected. If a pooled reagent with a single fluorochrome is used, negative results are obtained directly from the results of the pooled stain. If the pooled stain is positive, however, then individual stains must be done for each of the individual viruses included in the pool. There are now commercial reagents that are a pool of antibodies in which one antibody has a different fluorochrome than all the other antibodies. Millipore markets SimulFluor Pooled DFA reagent, which differentiates RSV from other viruses in the pool, and Diagnostic Hybrids markets the D3 Duet Respiratory Virus Screening Kits, which have differential staining for either influenza A or RSV in pooled reagents. This differentiation allows the specimens positive for the virus with the unique fluorochrome to be reported directly from the results of the pooled stain. Staining with pooled immunofluorescent reagents can result in a savings in labor, although this will depend on which viruses are present in the specimens a laboratory tests and the fraction of specimens that are negative for those viruses.

Shih and colleagues evaluated the utility of MDCK cells in shell-vial culture at 24 hours, and also determined the gain of testing an additional vial at 48 hours and the gain of using HEp-2 cells at 24 and 48 hours (**Table 1**).[18] Shell-vial cultures were stained with a commercial pool of antibodies, followed by staining with individual antibodies if the pool was positive (Bartels, WA, USA). The reference standard was conventional culture with MDCK, MK-2, MRC-5 and HEp-2 for up to 30 days. The

Table 1
Sensitivity of shell-vial cultures for respiratory viruses

Cell Lines	Screening Stain (Fluorescence Assay)	Days Stained	Influenza A %	Influenza B (%)	RSV (%)	Adenovirus (%)	Parainfluenza 1 (%)	Parainfluenza 2 (%)	Parainfluenza 3 (%)	References
MDCK	IFA, Bartels	1	81.5	26.7	82.6	79.6	100[a]	25[a]	73.3	Shih et al[18]
MDCK and A549	IFA, Bartels	3, 7	100	ND	72	66[a]	100[a]	100[a]	100[a]	Lee et al[19]
PMK and A549	IFA, Bartels	2, 3	94[b]							Matthey et al[20]
PMK and A549	IFA, Bartels	2	ND	94	75	83	33[a]	75[a]	79	Rabalais et al[21]

Abbreviation: ND, not determined because this virus was not detected in any specimens.
[a] Fewer than 10 specimens contained this virus.
[b] The data were pooled in the original report and so sensitivities for some viruses are indicated by combination of the columns.

use of an MDCK-shell vial at 24 hours was surprisingly sensitive (see **Table 1**) for most viruses, but it was insensitive for detection of influenza B viruses. Incubation of the MDCK for an additional 24 hours (48 hours total) more than doubled the number of influenza B-positive specimens detected, but this only raised the sensitivity to approximately half that of conventional tube culture.[18] The addition of HEp-2 cells increased the sensitivity for RSV from 82.6% to 100%, and also increased detection of parainfluenza viruses and adenoviruses, although only small numbers of these were detected in the study.[18]

One report suggests that the use of MDCK and A549 shell vials can be more sensitive than conventional culture for detection of some respiratory viruses (see **Table 1**).[19] Three and 7 days after initiation, shell-vial cultures were stained with a commercial pool of antibodies, followed by staining with individual antibodies if the pool was positive (Bartels, WA, USA). The reference standard was conventional culture with HEp-2 and PMK for 7 days. For all respiratory viruses analyzed, the sensitivity of the shell-vial culture was 81.9% versus 72.3% for conventional culture (calculations by the present authors, not included in the reference). The shell vials were more sensitive than conventional cultures for influenza A (100% and 42% respectively) and also detected a few more isolates of parainfluenza viruses, although the total number of parainfluenza viruses was small.[19] Conventional culture was more sensitive than shell-vial culture for RSV (86% and 72% respectively).

The use of PMK and A549 cells in shell-vial culture has been evaluated in two studies (see **Table 1**).[20,21] Rabalais and colleagues incubated shell vials for 3 days and stained with the same pooled antibody reagent as those discussed earlier, with staining with individual antibodies if the pool was positive (Bartels, WA, USA).[21] The reference standard was conventional culture with PMK, A549 and HEp-2 cells for up to 14 days. The overall sensitivity of the two methods was similar; shell vial detected 79% of all positive specimens, while conventional culture detected 80% of all positives specimens. Shell-vial culture results were complete in 2 days, while the results of conventional culture took a mean of 7.6 days, with a range of 1 to 14 days. The shell-vial culture was sensitive for influenza B virus, detecting more positive specimens than did conventional culture (no influenza A positive specimens were detected by either method). The two methods were of comparable sensitivity for RSV (75% for shell-vial culture, 70% for conventional culture, calculations by the present authors, not included in the reference). Although the methods were somewhat different, Matthey and colleagues reached similar conclusions, in that shell-vial culture had an overall high sensitivity (94%).[20] Out of 10 specimens positive for influenza A virus, 9 were detected by conventional culture and all 10 were detected by shell-vial culture.

A useful commercial product for shell-vial culture of respiratory viruses, R-Mix (Diagnostic Hybrids, Inc, Athens, Ohio), contains a mixture of a mink lung cell line (Mv1Lu) with A549 cells. Because the cell lines are combined in the same shell vial, fewer shell vials need to be used. The rationale for selecting these cell lines is that A549 should support replication of RSV, adenovirus and parainfluenza viruses, while Mv1Lu will support replication of influenza viruses. In practice, it appears that both the cell lines work well for each of the viruses.[22]

Several studies have been done to determine the sensitivity of R-Mix for detection of respiratory viruses (**Table 2**).[23–26] Each of these studies included some type of conventional culture in the reference standard, and some also included direct antigen testing,[24,26] or another shell-vial culture system.[23] Most studies found that R-Mix is sensitive for detection of influenza A and B viruses, with reported sensitivities of 89% to 98% and 94.7% to 100%, respectively.[24–26] In one study, the sensitivity for

Table 2
Sensitivity of R-Mix shell-vial cultures for respiratory viruses

Cell Lines	Screening Stain (FA)	Days Stained	Influenza A (%)	Influenza B (%)	RSV (%)	Adenovirus (%)	Parainfluenza 1 (%)	Parainfluenza 2 (%)	Parainfluenza 3 (%)	References
Mv1Lu and A549 (R-Mix)	D3, Diagnostic Hybrids	1, 2	78[a]		73	45	83[a]			LaSala et al[23]
Mv1Lu and A549 (R-Mix)	Pooled Reagent, Bartels	1, then CPE to 10 for HA	98.8	94.7	86.7	68.6	86.7	100[b]	83.3[b]	Dunn et al[24]
Mv1Lu and A549 (R-Mix)	None (Individual FA Used)	1, 2, 5	89[b]	100[b]	86	25	100[b]	80[b]	67	Weinberg et al[25]
Mv1Lu and A549 (R-Mix)	Respiratory Virus Screen, Chemicon	1	96	ND	ND	ND	ND	ND	ND	Fong et al[26]
Mv1Lu and A549 (R-Mix ReadyCells)	D3, Diagnostic Hybrids	1, 3	100	93	91	90	100			Kim et al[27]

Abbreviations: ND, not determined because this virus was not detected in any specimens; FA, Fluorescence assay.
[a] The data were pooled in the original report and so sensitivities for some viruses are indicated by combination of the columns.
[b] Fewer than ten specimens contained this virus.

influenza A and B (combined) was somewhat lower at 78%.[23] The reported sensitivity of R-Mix culture for RSV is moderate, with a range of 73.0% to 86.7%. Most of these studies did not include DFA in the gold standard for RSV, and since DFA is usually more sensitive than viral culture for RSV, they might overestimate the sensitivity of R-Mix culture. R-Mix has moderately low sensitivity for adenovirus, with a range of 25% to 68.6%. In each study where the comparison was made using fresh clinical specimens, the sensitivity of R-Mix for adenovirus was significantly lower than the sensitivity of conventional culture. Most studies did not include enough specimens with parainfluenza viruses to give a robust estimate of sensitivity, but in general R-Mix appears to be reasonably sensitive for these viruses. The combined sensitivity for parainfluenzas 1, 2 and 3 was 83% in one study,[23] and separate studies found sensitivities of 87.6% and 67% for parainfluenzas 1 and 3, respectively.[24,25]

A major advantage of R-Mix shell vials is the shorter turn-around time for positive and negative results. The time to detection of viruses is shorter with R-Mix than with conventional culture. LaSala and colleagues found that the mean time to detection of influenza virus was 1.1 days and 4.3 days for R-Mix and conventional culture, respectively.[23] For RSV, these authors found that the mean time to detection was 1.6 days and 10.2 days for R-Mix and conventional culture, respectively. The time to issue a negative report for R-Mix viral culture will depend on the days on which the shell vials are stained. Practice varies between the published studies, but in most studies the shell vial culture was complete within 3 days,[23,26] but some do hold them as long as 5 to 10 days.[24,25] In our laboratory, we stain R-Mix shell vials at 24 and 48 hours, allowing a maximum turn-around time of 2 days. Cryopreserved R-Mix shell vials with a shelf life of up to 6 months are also available. These shell vials have been validated in one study (see **Table 2**).[27] They are reported to have a high sensitivity for influenza viruses, RSV, adenovirus, and parainfluenza viruses when analyzed on day 3.

The practice of using R-Mix shell-vial culture along with an additional shell vial with PMK has been evaluated.[28] These authors harvested R-Mix after a minimum of 20 hours incubation, and performed terminal HA on PMK shell vials after 10 to 14 days. Ninety-five percent of influenza A and B, and parainfluenza types 1, 2 and 3 were detected by R-Mix and only an additional 5% were detected by the terminal HA.[28] The detection of a small number of additional positives at 10 to 14 days is of limited value. R-Mix culture alone was adequate, at least for the HA positive viruses.

SUMMARY

Recently there have been several important improvements in viral culture. MDCK-SIAT1 cells are a useful addition to the available cell lines for influenza viral culture. They can be used in an accurate bioassay for the response of influenza isolates to neuraminidase inhibitors, and also show promise for use in detection of influenza viruses from clinical specimens. HuH7 cells are another promising cell line for use in viral culture for respiratory viruses, although definitive data supporting the use of these is needed. Shell-vial culture is a sensitive method for detection of respiratory viruses. An important advantage of shell-vial culture is the markedly reduced turn-around time for the culture. While shell vials containing a single cell line can be used to detect respiratory viruses, the total number of shell vials needed, and the labor of the culture, can be reduced using commercial R-Mix shell vials, which have a combination of two cell lines. This combination allows a single type of shell vial to be used for respiratory virus culture.

REFERENCES

1. Washington W, Allen S, Janda W, et al. Koneman's color atlas and textbook of diagnostic microbioloty. Baltimore (MD): Lippincott Williams and Wilkins; 2006.
2. Nicholls JM, Chan RW, Russell RJ, et al. Evolving complexities of influenza virus and its receptors. Trends Microbiol 2008;16(4):149–57.
3. Matrosovich M, Matrosovich T, Carr J, et al. Overexpression of the alpha-2,6-sialyltransferase in MDCK cells increases influenza virus sensitivity to neuraminidase inhibitors. J Virol 2003;77(15):8418–25.
4. Dharan NJ, Gubareva LV, Meyer JJ, et al. Infections with oseltamivir-resistant influenza A(H1N1) virus in the United States. JAMA 2009;301(10):1034–41.
5. Hatakeyama S, Sakai-Tagawa Y, Kiso M, et al. Enhanced expression of an alpha2,6-linked sialic acid on MDCK cells improves isolation of human influenza viruses and evaluation of their sensitivity to a neuraminidase inhibitor. J Clin Microbiol 2005;43(8):4139–46.
6. Oh DY, Barr IG, Mosse JA, et al. MDCK-SIAT1 cells show improved isolation rates for recent human influenza viruses compared to conventional MDCK cells. J Clin Microbiol 2008;46(7):2189–94.
7. Keskinen P, Nyqvist M, Sareneva T, et al. Impaired antiviral response in human hepatoma cells. Virology 1999;263(2):364–75.
8. Freymuth F, Vabret A, Rozenberg F, et al. Replication of respiratory viruses, particularly influenza virus, rhinovirus, and coronavirus in HuH7 hepatocarcinoma cell line. J Med Virol 2005;77(2):295–301.
9. Pene F, Merlat A, Vabret A, et al. Coronavirus 229E-related pneumonia in immunocompromised patients. Clin Infect Dis 2003;37(7):929–32.
10. Tang BS, Chan KH, Cheng VC, et al. Comparative host gene transcription by microarray analysis early after infection of the Huh7 cell line by severe acute respiratory syndrome coronavirus and human coronavirus 229E. J Virol 2005;79(10):6180–93.
11. Johnston SL, Siegel CS. A comparison of direct immunofluorescence, shell vial culture, and conventional cell culture for the rapid detection of influenza A and B. Diagn Microbiol Infect Dis 1991;14(2):131–4.
12. Espy MJ, Smith TF, Harmon MW, et al. Rapid detection of influenza virus by shell vial assay with monoclonal antibodies. J Clin Microbiol 1986;24(4):677–9.
13. Reina J, Fernandez-Baca V, Blanco I, et al. Comparison of Madin-Darby canine kidney cells (MDCK) with a green monkey continuous cell line (Vero) and human lung embryonated cells (MRC-5) in the isolation of influenza A virus from nasopharyngeal aspirates by shell vial culture. J Clin Microbiol 1997;35(7):1900–1.
14. Meqdam MM, Nasrallah GK. Enhanced detection of respiratory syncytial virus by shell vial in children hospitalised with respiratory illnesses in northern Jordan. J Med Virol 2000;62(4):518–23.
15. Pedneault L, Robillard L, Turgeon JP. Validation of respiratory syncytial virus enzyme immunoassay and shell vial assay results. J Clin Microbiol 1994;32(11):2861–4.
16. Smith MC, Creutz C, Huang YT. Detection of respiratory syncytial virus in nasopharyngeal secretions by shell vial technique. J Clin Microbiol 1991;29(3):463–5.
17. Johnston SL, Siegel CS. Evaluation of direct immunofluorescence, enzyme immunoassay, centrifugation culture, and conventional culture for the detection of respiratory syncytial virus. J Clin Microbiol 1990;28(11):2394–7.

18. Shih SR, Tsao KC, Ning HC, et al. Diagnosis of respiratory tract viruses in 24 h by immunofluorescent staining of shell vial cultures containing Madin-Darby Canine Kidney (MDCK) cells. J Virol Methods 1999;81(1–2):77–81.
19. Lee SH, Boutilier JE, MacDonald MA, et al. Enhanced detection of respiratory viruses using the shell vial technique and monoclonal antibodies. J Virol Methods 1992;39(1–2):39–46.
20. Matthey S, Nicholson D, Ruhs S, et al. Rapid detection of respiratory viruses by shell vial culture and direct staining by using pooled and individual monoclonal antibodies. J Clin Microbiol 1992;30(3):540–4.
21. Rabalais GP, Stout GG, Ladd KL, et al. Rapid diagnosis of respiratory viral infections by using a shell vial assay and monoclonal antibody pool. J Clin Microbiol 1992;30(6):1505–8.
22. Huang YT, Turchek BM. Mink lung cells and mixed mink lung and A549 cells for rapid detection of influenza virus and other respiratory viruses. J Clin Microbiol 2000;38(1):422–3.
23. LaSala PR, Bufton KK, Ismail N, et al. Prospective comparison of R-mix shell vial system with direct antigen tests and conventional cell culture for respiratory virus detection. J Clin Virol 2007;38(3):210–6.
24. Dunn JJ, Woolstenhulme RD, Langer J, et al. Sensitivity of respiratory virus culture when screening with R-mix fresh cells. J Clin Microbiol 2004;42(1):79–82.
25. Weinberg A, Brewster L, Clark J, et al. Evaluation of R-Mix shell vials for the diagnosis of viral respiratory tract infections. J Clin Virol 2004;30(1):100–5.
26. Fong CK, Lee MK, Griffith BP. Evaluation of R-Mix FreshCells in shell vials for detection of respiratory viruses. J Clin Microbiol 2000;38(12):4660–2.
27. Kim JS, Kim SH, Bae SY, et al. Enhanced detection of respiratory viruses using cryopreserved R-Mix ReadyCells. J Clin Virol 2008;42(3):264–7.
28. Taggart EW, Crist G, Billetdeaux E, et al. Utility of terminal hemadsorption for detection of hemadsorbing respiratory viruses from conventional shell vial cultures for laboratories using R-Mix cultures. J Clin Virol 2009;44(1):86–7.

Developments in Immunologic Assays for Respiratory Viruses

Marie Louise Landry, MD[a,b],*

KEYWORDS

- Respiratory viruses • Immunoassay
- Influenza virus • Respiratory syncytial virus
- Immunofluorescence • Lateral flow assay

For 50 years, virus isolation using conventional cell cultures has been considered the gold standard for the diagnosis of respiratory viruses. However, the time to result for some viruses can be a week or more, and the expertise and facilities are not available in many hospitals. Molecular amplification methods for respiratory viruses are increasing in availability, but are expensive and often require transport to a reference laboratory. Results usually require 1 to 3 days, even when done on site, and the effect on clinical care is uncertain.

Immunologic assays use antibodies to detect viral antigens directly in clinical samples, and are the most rapid and least expensive of the available test options. The development of monoclonal antibody (MAb) technology significantly improved the availability and consistency of immunoassays. They require from 10 minutes to a few hours to complete, can be done multiple times a day, and some can be performed around the clock and at the point of care. Consequently, in most hospitals, clinics, and doctor's offices, immunologic assays are the only tests performed on site for the diagnosis of respiratory viruses. In most cases, testing is limited to influenza types A and B and respiratory syncytial virus (RSV), the most common respiratory viruses, and the only respiratory viruses with approved antiviral therapies.

In hospitalized patients, rapid immunologic assays facilitate infection control measures, bed management, and cohorting of patients with the same infection. More than other methods, immunoassays have been shown to affect patient management including early administration of antiviral therapy, reduction in unnecessary tests

[a] Department of Laboratory Medicine, Yale University School of Medicine, PO Box 208035, 333 Cedar Street, New Haven, CT 06520-8035, USA
[b] Department of Laboratory Medicine, Yale New Haven Hospital, Clinical Virology Laboratory, New Haven, 20 York Street, CT 06504, USA
* Department of Laboratory Medicine, Yale University School of Medicine, PO Box 208035, 333 Cedar Street, New Haven, CT 06520-8035.
E-mail address: marie.landry@yale.edu

Clin Lab Med 29 (2009) 635–647
doi:10.1016/j.cll.2009.07.003
0272-2712/09/$ – see front matter © 2009 Elsevier Inc. All rights reserved.

labmed.theclinics.com

and antibiotics, and earlier discharges.[1–4] Thus, immunoassays remain essential components of the diagnostic armamentarium.

This article discusses the major immunologic methods employed for respiratory virus diagnosis, recent developments in immunoassays and sample collection, and current test algorithms.

IMMUNOLOGIC METHODS
Immunofluorescence

Immunofluorescence (IF) techniques have long been used for the diagnosis of viral diseases. The method was introduced by Albert Coons and colleagues in 1941,[5,6] and was first applied to the direct detection of influenza A in nasal smears in 1956.[6] In the 1980s, IF was applied to RSV,[7] parainfluenza,[8,9] and adenovirus[10] diagnosis, and recently to human metapneumovirus (HMPV).[11] Initially, obtaining a dependable supply of high-quality, specific, polyclonal antibodies was difficult and testing was confined to a few laboratories. Indeed, the goal of sharing high-quality IF reagents and protocols was the major impetus for the founding of the European and Pan American Groups for Rapid Viral Diagnosis.[12] High-quality commercial MAbs have brought IF within the reach of all virology laboratories.

IF requires more technical expertise than other immunologic methods. It is labor intensive, manual, and operator dependent, and requires a substantial, sustained commitment on the part of the results are highly variable from laboratory to laboratory. Yet when done well, IF is the most sensitive and specific immunoassay, able to detect just one infected cell. IF is also the only current immunologic method that can screen for 7 to 8 viruses in a single assay.[13] Adequate ciliated respiratory epithelial cells (Fig. 1A) are essential for valid results.

Nasopharyngeal or mid-turbinate samples, but not throat swabs, are good sources for ciliated cells. It is not uncommon for 10% or more of samples upon final examination of the stained slide to be rated inadequate because of insufficient cells (<20–25 cells per slide). IF performs best in settings where sample quality can be improved through direct feedback and training.

Direct or indirect IF procedures can be used. In the direct fluorescent antibody (DFA) procedure, a fluorescent dye is directly conjugated to the specific antibody. DFA is quicker, simpler and exhibits less nonspecific staining. The indirect fluorescent antibody (IFA) procedure uses a specific primary antibody that is not conjugated but is

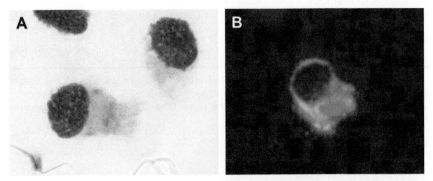

Fig. 1. (A) Ciliated respiratory epithelial cell, Wright's stain. (B) Ciliated respiratory epithelial cell showing intracytoplasmic staining with a fluorescein-labeled anti-HMPV MAb.

allowed to react with the test antigen. Then fluorescent-conjugated antibody, directed against the animal species from which the primary antibody is made, is added. IFA is sometimes more sensitive than DFA, but requires additional incubation and wash steps, and gives more nonspecific results. In general, clinical laboratories prefer the DFA protocol when available.

Standard IF steps include (1) centrifuge samples to pellet the cells, (2) wash the cells to remove mucus if needed, (3) apply cell pellets to slides by pipette or cytocentrifuge, (4) dry the slide, (5) fix the cells in acetone, (6) apply fluorophore labeled antibodies, (7) incubate in a humidified chamber to allow the antibodies to bind, (8) wash to remove unreacted reagents, (9) apply mounting reagent and a coverslip, and finally (10) examine the entire slide by fluorescence microscopy.

IF on clinical specimens is more challenging than IF on cell cultures, and partnering with an experienced laboratory, exchanging slides, saving slides for 2 to 4 weeks at 4°C until culture results are completed to allow re-examination if needed, are recommended.

To obtain accurate results, labeled intracellular antigen in a distribution (intracytoplasmic or intranuclear) expected for the particular virus (see **Fig. 1**B) must be distinguished from nonspecific fluorescence seen with bacteria, fungi, and mucus. A regularly serviced fluorescence microscope with high-quality objectives and a bright bulb, housed in a dark room, is essential or samples with few positive cells may be missed. Solutions for the technical problems that can be encountered have recently been reviewed.[14]

Originally, separate cell spots and antibodies were required for each virus, and tests were selectively performed based on the most prevalent circulating viruses. In 1998, 2-virus MAb pools became commercially available for direct staining of respiratory viruses, followed in 2000 by 7-virus MAb pools (**Table 1**). A respiratory virus screen reagent can be applied to a single cell spot to detect 7 viruses (RSV, influenza A and B, parainfluenza types 1, 2, 3, and adenovirus) year-round.[13] This multiplex approach is similar to culture, and dual infections can be detected. Multiplex DFA can detect more viruses, even in samples from adults, than a commonly used rapid test for influenza (**Table 2**).[15] Recently, MAbs to HMPV have become available, and have been incorporated into dual and pooled reagents.[11,16]

Using two different fluorophore labels has also made diagnosis more efficient. For dual-target reagents, each of the two antibodies has a different fluorescent label, and in pools of 7 antibodies, the most commonly sought virus (RSV or influenza A) can be labeled with rhodamine (orange-gold) or phycoerythrin (yellow); the remaining viral antibodies are labeled with fluorescein (apple-green). When cells fluoresce apple-green, identification of the specific virus requires either staining two additional slides with dual reagents or spotting cells onto a microscope slide and staining with individual MAbs. Rhodamine and phycoerythrin fluorescence can be seen with the fluorescein filter, although rhodamine staining is brighter when a second rhodamine filter is used.

Cytospin preparation of slides to enhance cell recovery and morphology was first used for cytomegalovirus (CMV) antigenemia,[17] then for herpes simplex virus (HSV) DFA,[18] and subsequently for respiratory samples.[13,19] Cytospin preparation gives fewer inadequate slides and greater sensitivity and specificity. In the author's laboratory, the sensitivity of cytospin DFA compared with conventional culture for adult and pediatric patients combined is consistently greater than 95% for RSV and seasonal influenza, greater than 90% for parainfluenza, but only 60% to 70% for adenovirus. From the first 400 Novel H1N1 (swine-origin) influenza viruses detected in the author's laboratory, cytospin DFA detected 82% to 85% compared with 45 cycles

Table 1
Immunological methods for diagnosis of respiratory virus infections

Method	Viruses Detected	Assay Time[a]	Frequency of Testing	Equipment	Expertise Required	Sensitivity/ Specificity[b]	Comments
Immunofluorescence using single antibody and fluorescein label; or pool of 2 to 8 MAbs, with two different fluorescent labels	RSV, Influenza A, Influenza B, parainfluenza types 1, 2, 3, adenovirus, HMPV	Standard protocol: 1.5–2 hrs Liquid staining: 40 min	On demand or batched several times a day	Centrifuge Cytospin (optional) Fluorescence microscope	Substantial	60–99%/96–100% Varies with virus, reagents, lab protocol, and operator	Samples may have insufficient cilliated cells for testing Cytospin slide preparation increases cell count and reading accuracy
ELISA, microwell	HMPV	1 hr	Batched once a day	ELISA washer and reader	Moderate	No data	Research use only in United States
ELISA, membrane casseette	RSV Influenza A Influenza A & B	30 min	On demand	None	Minimal	40%–90%/ 96%–100%	Requires serial timed additions of reagents and washes.

Method	Targets	Time				Sensitivity/Specificity	Comments
Lateral flow immunochromatography[c], visual read	RSV, Influenza A & B	15 min	On demand	None	Minimal	40%-90%/100%	Requires addition of sample only
	H5N1[d]	40 min	On demand	None	Moderate	No H5N1 patient studies	Two-step protocol
Lateral flow, with reader	RSV, Influenza A & B, Influenza A & B, plus H1, H3 subtype	15 min	On demand	Reader	Minimal	70%-100% 98%-100%	Reader provides objective interpretation & print-out

[a] Includes sample preparation.
[b] Samples containing high titers of virus give best results. Comparator assay is usually convertional or rapid culture. Quality and performance of comparator assays is suboptimal in some studies.
[c] Several assays are CLIA waived.
[d] AVantage TM A/H5N1 Flu Test kit was approved by the FDA in April, 2009 for use only in high complexity laboratories. A series of 3 reagents must be added to the sample before it is added to the test cassette. Clinical trials were done on patients with possible seasonal influenza (H5N1 negative) and cell culture isolates (H5N1 positive).

Data from Landry ML, Ferguson D. Suboptimal detection of influenza virus in adults by the Directigen Flu A1B enzyme immunoassay and correlation of results with the number of antigen-positive cells detected by cytospin immunofluorescence. J Clin Microbiol 2003;41:3407–9.

Table 2
Comparison of a rapid influenza test and cytospin-enhanced respiratory virus screen DFA in NP swabs from adults

Virus	No. Detected by Method (N = 152)	
	Rapid Test	Respiratory Virus Screen DFA
Influenza A	16	31
Influenza B	0	0
RSV	NA	3
Parainfluenza 1,2,3	NA	1
Adenovirus	NA	2
Total no. detected	16	37

Abbreviation: NA, not available.
Data from Ref.[15]

of real-time polymerase chain reaction (PCR) (http://www.who.int/csr/resources/publications/swineflu/realtimeptpcr).

A disadvantage of DFA is the total assay time of 1.5 to 2 hours compared with the 10 to 30 minutes required for rapid tests. A new IF strategy uses a liquid format to detect 8 viruses within 10 minutes of obtaining the cell pellet. The D³ Ultra Duet procedure (Diagnostic Hybrids Inc, Athens, OH) uses a proprietary reagent to permeabilize the cells in a liquid suspension, and allows antibodies with fluorescent dye molecules access into the cells. After a 5-minute incubation, the cells are rinsed, centrifuged for 2 minutes and loaded onto a proprietary slide. The D³ Ultra Duet assays use two different fluorophores in 3 pairs of MAb combinations: FluA/Flu B; RSV/HMPV; Para 1,2,3/Adenovirus. The 3 MAb combinations for each sample are separately incubated, then centrifuged and finally applied to separate wells of a slide for examination.[16]

IF has revolutionized culture methods by permitting the rapid identification of cell culture isolates once cytopathic effects develop, and the early detection of virus replication in cultures after only 1 to 2 days of incubation and before cyto-pathic effects appear.[20]

Other IF innovations, not yet used for respiratory virus diagnosis, include automated instruments to add reagents and wash slides, and image analysis using computer software to automate slide reading.[14,21] IF is a versatile technique that can detect multiple viruses in a short period of time, can be done on demand when the virology laboratory is open, and can provide sensitive and specific results provided the laboratory is highly committed and detail-oriented.

Enzyme-Linked Immunosorbent Assay

In 1971, Engvall and Perlmann introduced the enzyme-linked immunosorbent assay (ELISA).[22] ELISA for antigen detection traditionally uses an antibody bound to a solid phase such as a microwell, tube, or bead to capture the antigens in the sample. A second enzyme-labeled detection antibody is then added. After washing away unreacted reagents, a substrate is added and, if the enzyme-labeled antibody is bound to viral antigens, a visible color reaction occurs that can be read visually or quantitated using a spectrophotometer. Whereas IF detects only viral proteins in infected cells, ELISA can also detect cell-free viral proteins. Additional advantages include ability to automate and an objective printed read-out. Microwell ELISA is often batched once a day and assay time is 1 to 3 hours.

In the 1980s, microwell ELISA was first applied to detection of respiratory viruses, RSV[23,24] and influenza A.[25] Although a-microwell ELISA for HMPV has recently been developed (Biotrin International, Dublin, Ireland), the microwell format in the United States has largely been replaced by other methods.

Membrane ELISA using individual cassettes, requiring no equipment and only 20 to 30 minutes to complete, comprised the first generation of rapid tests for RSV and influenza. Since membrane ELISAs require a series of timed reagent additions, incubations and wash steps, the addition of the substrate and finally a stop reagent-, they are considered moderately complex by Clinical Laboratory Improvement Amendments (CLIA) and must be done in a laboratory. Current examples include Directigen RSV and Directigen Flu A+B kits.

Membrane ELISAs for RSV have been successful in pediatric populations, because of the high titers of virus shed and the insensitivity and slowness of conventional culture methods. ELISAs for RSV and influenza have not been so successful in adults, who shed lower titers of virus.[15,26,27] In general, nonamplified immunoassays require 100,000 or more viral particles for a positive result. With all ELISAs, careful and thorough washing is critical or false positives can occur. For membrane assays, viscous samples such as nasopharyngeal (NP) aspirates can trap reagents and give false-positive results.

Lateral Flow Immunochromatography

Advances in antiviral therapy for influenza made rapid and accessible diagnostic tests a high priority. Neuraminidase inhibitors must be started within 48 hours of symptom onset to have an effect.[28] Thus rapid-influenza tests that could be completed within less than 15 minutes and used at the point of care (POC) in the clinic or emergency department (ED) were introduced. One of the earliest tests, QuickVue, used lateral flow immunochromatography (LFIC)[29] and over the past decade numerous tests using LFIC have been approved by the US Food and Drug Administration (FDA). In addition to QuickVue Influenza A+B, examples include BinaxNOW Influenza A&B, Directigen EZ Flu A+B, OSOM Influenza A&B, SAS FLUAlert, TRU FLU, and Xpect Flu A&B kits. For a list of current FDA-approved rapid influenza tests, see the Centers for Disease Control and Prevention (CDC) Web site (http://www.cdc.gov/flu/professionals/diagnosis/labprocedures.htm). Similar tests for RSV are available from most of the manufacturers of rapid influenza tests.

By LFIC, an antibody specific for the target is immobilized on a membrane (**Fig. 2**). A detector reagent, usually an antibody coupled to colloidal gold, is deposited onto the conjugate pad. When a sample is added to the conjugate pad, the detector reagent is solubilized and begins to move with sample flow along the membrane strip. Virus in the sample binds to the detector reagent, and as it passes over the capture reagent, the antigen-antibody-colloidal gold complex is trapped, and a color appears in proportion to the amount of antigen. LFIC assays can be a strip affixed to a card, a strip held within a plastic cassette, or a strip inserted into the sample solution. Samples can be a swab eluted into a buffer, an aspirate, or a wash. In contrast to ELISA, with LFIC the sample is simply added to the strip, or the test strip is inserted into the sample solution, and the timer is set. Yet performance is similar to membrane ELISA.[30,31]

For optimal performance, it is essential that the manufacturer's instructions for sample type, collection device, and preparation are carefully followed. Although a few kits allow a variety of viral transport media, many kits require use of their own device, and if other tests such as IF, culture or PCR are performed, a second sample must be collected. If only a rapid test is done, using the smallest volume of recommended media or buffer concentrates the sample and gives a better result. Multipurpose

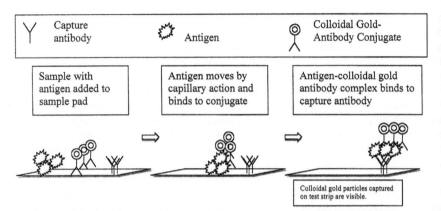

Fig. 2. Lateral flow immunochromatography for viral antigen detection. (*Reproduced from* Campbell S, Landry ML. Rapid antigen tests. In: Tang, Y-W, Stratton, CW, editors. Advanced techniques in diagnostic microbiology. New YorK: Springer; 2006. p. 28; with permission.)

viral transport media, in 2 to 3 mL volume, allow multiple tests to be performed on one sample, but dilute the sample.

As with ELISA, 10^4 to 10^5 or more viral particles are generally needed for a positive result. Thus, for a more definitive answer, samples with negative rapid test results should be tested by culture or PCR. Efforts to improve the sensitivity of lateral flow assays are ongoing. In recent studies, the new fluorescent-based 3M test has been reported to be more sensitive than first-generation LFIC assays for influenza and RSV.[32,33]

Specificity may be more of a concern with the simple rapid tests, especially at times of low disease prevalence when false positives can exceed true positives. Whereas nonspecific IF staining patterns can be differentiated microscopically by an expert reader, the same is not true for ELISA and lateral flow tests. Thus, these tests should be confined to periods of high prevalence and to patients with compatible symptoms (http://www.cdc.gov/flu/professionals/diagnosis/labprocedures.htm).

Test performance in published studies may not be replicated in practice.[34] This can often be attributed to better sample collection in studies, use of predominantly pediatric samples, or suboptimal performance of the comparator method caused by sample freezing or shipping of samples to a reference laboratory and delayed inoculation into culture. For influenza, seasonal antigenic variation can affect testing. Several studies have found reduced sensitivity for detection of influenza B.[35,36] The variation in published results underscores the need for laboratories to perform an in-house comparison with their existing methods whenever possible. How well rapid tests perform with Novel H1N1 (swine-origin) influenza has not yet been established.

Simple rapid influenza tests have made it feasible for all hospitals to have testing on site. Rapid results are useful for infection control measures and initiating antivirals, and are the only tests available around the clock.[37] A study in a pediatric ED showed that results available on the chart when doctors see the patients improve patient management and save costs.[3] In addition, rapid-influenza tests have had a major impact on influenza surveillance.

Of current tests, only 3 have been waived by CLIA. Although they are simple tests, more errors occur when performed by nonlaboratory personnel.[38,39] Training and monitoring of personnel competence are essential for accurate results. If personnel do not read the test strips promptly at the end of the incubation, erroneous results may be obtained. To avoid this, the 3M test, recently approved by the FDA, uses an automated reader that prints the results at the end of the incubation. The reader can be linked to the laboratory information system to reduce labor and avoid transcription errors.[32,33]

Another new lateral flow POC test, fluID, determines influenza A and B and subtypes H1 and H3. Like 3M, fluID uses fluorescence and an objective reader to increase accuracy.[40] To improve sensitivity of detection, fluID technology uses highly specific and efficient binding pairs made up of pRNA, a synthetic reagent designed to yield high binding affinities at room temperature. The detection reagent is analyte-specific MAb bound to highly fluorescent polystyrene microbeads. A swab is dipped into a device containing extraction reagents, which is then inserted into the test cartridge. Finally the test cartridge is inserted into a low-cost portable fluorescence detection reader. Results from preclinical studies show higher sensitivities than first-generation lateral flow assays.[40]

In April, 2009, the FDA approved a lateral flow assay for avian influenza H5N1, AVantage A/H5N1 Flu Test, for use only in high complexity laboratories. The test uses a combination of gold-conjugated pan-reactive monoclonal anti-influenza A antibodies and recombinant proteins containing the PDZ domains to capture the nonstructural protein 1 (NS1) from H5N1. The test is intended for swabs collected in M4 transport media and requires addition of three reagents to the sample (lysis buffer, loading buffer, and detector reagent) before adding the solution to the sample well of the test cassette. Results are interpreted visually by the presence, absence, and relative intensity of color lines on the membrane. Clinical trials were limited to patient samples collected during the influenza season (H5N1 negative) and culture isolates of H5N1. The performance of the test with clinical specimens from humans infected with H5N1 influenza viruses has not been established. More details about AVantage can be found at http://www.accessdata.fda.gov/cdrh_docs/reviews/K083278.pdf.

Table 3
Recent developments in immunologic assays for respiratory viruses

Immunofluorescence	Microwell ELISA	Rapid Influenza and RSV Tests	Sample Collection
Dual fluorophores for efficient identification	HMPV kit (research use only in United States)	Lateral flow assays that require addition of sample only	Special collection devices for some kits
Pooled antibodies for multiplex screening of 2–8 viruses		Approval of POC tests Automated reader for lateral flow assay to provide objective read-out and permanent record	Low volume collection media to minimize dilution Flocked swabs to increase virus and cells in test sample
Cytospin slide preparation to improve sensitivity and specificity		Lateral flow assay to subtype influenza for seasonal H1 and H3	Mid-turbinate sample to improve collection and patient acceptance
HMPV commercial DFA reagents			Self-collected samples to facilitate surveillance and diagnosis
Liquid staining of cells to shorten assay time from 90 to 40 min			

Table 4
Use of immunoassays in respiratory virus diagnosis

Setting	Sample	Test
Doctor's office	Upper respiratory	Rapid test
ED or hospital clinic	Upper respiratory	Rapid test or DFA
Hospitalized patient, normal host	Upper respiratory	Rapid test or DFA, optional reflex to culture or PCR if result negative
Hospitalized patient, compromised host or severe illness	Upper respiratory	Rapid test or DFA, plus culture or PCR
Inpatient or outpatient	Lower respiratory	Rapid test or DFA, plus culture or PCR

SAMPLE TYPE AND COLLECTION DEVICE

Whereas culture and molecular amplification methods amplify input virus, immunoassays do not. Therefore optimal sample collection is even more important. IF requires abundant ciliated respiratory epithelial cells (the target cells for viral replication), and ELISA and lateral flow assays require 100,000 virus particles or more. Training in sample collection and use of trained collectors, including respiratory therapists, will provide superior results.

Collection of samples early in illness is recommended, when virus shedding is maximal. However, a recent study has found that within the first 12 hours after symptom onset, virus shedding may be low and rapid tests falsely negative.[41] The author has also observed very early samples that are negative by IF, while samples collected from the same patients 8 hours later are strongly positive.

NP aspirates and washes have long been considered the best sample type, but collection of swabs is simpler, more acceptable (especially to adults), and is gaining wider acceptance. When the test is done properly, results can be comparable. To reach the nasopharynx requires deep insertion of the swab, so NP swabs often have a flexible wire shaft with a small tip for comfort. However, the small surface area can lead to inadequate cell collection; a larger-tipped swab with a more rigid shaft is an alternative used in the author's laboratory. Collection from the mid-turbinate region of the nose, which has abundant ciliated epithelial cells, is more comfortable for the patient. Throat swabs alone have been judged inferior for recovery of respiratory viruses and provide many fewer ciliated cells for DFA.

Recently, flocked swabs have been introduced which have an open structure, act like a soft brush, and more efficiently release sample into the transport media than traditional mattress swabs. Several studies have shown flocked swabs to be superior to traditional swabs and comparable to aspirates in yield, yet less invasive, more acceptable for the patient, and less prone to producing aerosols than aspirates.[42,43]

SUMMARY

Immunoassays are the most commonly used tests for the diagnosis of respiratory viruses. Continued improvements have kept them relevant and useful (**Table 3**).

IF was the first immunoassay applied to respiratory virus diagnosis and continuing improvements have increased its utility. Although IF requires substantial commitment and attention to detail, it can be performed by any virology laboratory experienced in IF for cell culture identification. On-site virus isolation also provides an essential foundation and comparator method to develop IF expertise and help monitor test performance.

MAb pools that detect up to 8 viruses and use of two fluorescent labels allow efficient multiplex testing. Cytospin preparation of slides enhances sensitivity through increased cell yield and improved cell morphology. A proprietary, new, rapid, liquid staining method promises to reduce assay time. Future innovations may include automation through instruments that perform staining and washing, and image analysis programs that scan and interpret cell fluorescence.

Because of their rapid turnaround times, immunoassays are often performed as first-line tests on hospitalized patients, while culture or PCR results are pending (**Table 4**). IF and rapid respiratory virus tests have been shown to affect patient care and provide cost savings in pediatric populations. However, further work is needed to determine the costs and benefits of various test algorithms in different outpatient and inpatient settings and patient populations.

Limitations of simple rapid tests such as membrane ELISA and lateral flow assays are suboptimal sensitivity and specificity, and a test menu limited to influenza and RSV. Obtaining better samples through training of collectors and improved collection devices is well worth the effort. Recent developments in POC tests include improved sensitivity and specificity through novel fluorescent-based strategies with automated readers that provide objective read-outs and, once the sample is loaded, free the health care worker to pursue other tasks while not jeopardizing the accuracy of the result by delayed reading.

Although immunoassays target conserved proteins, antigenic variation between viral strains or between seasons can occur, leading to an unanticipated drop in assay sensitivity. However, immunoassays are the most rapid and economical of existing methods, and 50 years after their first application to respiratory viruses, continued improvements have kept them at the forefront of patient care.

REFERENCES

1. Poehling KA, Zhu Y, Tang YW, et al. Accuracy and impact of a point-of-care rapid influenza test in young children with respiratory illnesses. Arch Pediatr Adolesc Med 2006;160:713–8.
2. Barenfanger J, Drake C, Leon N, et al. Clinical and financial benefits of rapid detection of respiratory viruses: an outcomes study. J Clin Microbiol 2000;38:2824–8.
3. Bonner AB, Monroe KW, Talley LI, et al. Impact of the rapid diagnosis of influenza on physician decision-making and patient management in the pediatric emergency department: results of a randomized, prospective, controlled trial. Pediatrics 2003;112:363–7.
4. Woo PC, Chiu SS, Seto WH, et al. Cost-effectiveness of rapid diagnosis of viral respiratory tract infections in pediatric patients. J Clin Microbiol 1997;35:1579–81.
5. Coons AH, Creech HJ, Jones RN. Immunological properties of an antibody containing a fluorescent group. Proc Soc Exp Biol Med 1941;47:200–2.
6. Liu C. Rapid diagnosis of human influenza infection from nasal smears by means of fluorescein-labeled antibody. Proc Soc Exp Biol Med 1956;92:883–7.
7. Bell DM, Walsh EE, Hruska JF, et al. Rapid detection of respiratory syncytial virus with a monoclonal antibody. J Clin Microbiol 1983;17:1099–101.
8. Wong DT, Welliver RC, Riddlesberger KR, et al. Rapid diagnosis of parainfluenza virus infection in children. J Clin Microbiol 1982;16:164–7.

9. Waner JL, Whitehurst NJ, Downs T, et al. Production of monoclonal antibodies against parainfluenza 3 virus and their use in diagnosis by immunofluorescence. J Clin Microbiol 1985;22:535–8.
10. Kalter SS, Armour V, Reinarz JA. Rapid diagnosis of respiratory disease due to adenovirus and mycoplasma. Arch Gesamte Virusforsch 1969;28:34–40.
11. Landry ML, Cohen S, Ferguson D. Prospective study of human metapneumovirus detection in clinical samples by use of light diagnostics direct immunofluorescence reagent and real-time PCR. J Clin Microbiol 2008;46:1098–100.
12. Gardner PS, McQuillin J. Rapid virus diagnosis. 2nd edition. London, UK: Butterworths & Co; 1980.
13. Landry ML, Ferguson D. SimulFluor respiratory screen for rapid detection of multiple respiratory viruses in clinical specimens by immunofluorescence staining. J Clin Microbiol 2000;38:708–11.
14. Schutzbank TE, McGuire R, Scholl DR. Immunofluorescence. In: Specter S, Hodinka RL, Young SA, et al, editors. Clinical virology manual. 4th edition. Washington, DC: ASM Press; 2009. p. 77–88.
15. Landry ML, Ferguson D. Suboptimal detection of influenza virus in adults by the Directigen Flu A+B enzyme immunoassay and correlation of results with the number of antigen-positive cells detected by cytospin immunofluorescence. J Clin Microbiol 2003;41:3407–9.
16. Crowell M, Baalman N. Evaluation of the diagnostic hybrids D3 Ultra Duet respiratory virus identification kit for the detection of respiratory viruses directly from clinical specimens. In: 25th annual clinical virology symposium. Daytona Beach (FL); 2009.
17. Landry ML, Ferguson D. Comparison of quantitative cytomegalovirus antigenemia assay with culture methods and correlation with clinical disease. J Clin Microbiol 1993;31:2851–6.
18. Landry ML, Ferguson D, Wlochowski J. Detection of herpes simplex virus in clinical specimens by cytospin-enhanced direct immunofluorescence. J Clin Microbiol 1997;35:302–4.
19. Doing KM, Jerkofsky MA, Dow EG, et al. Use of fluorescent-antibody staining of cytocentrifuge-prepared smears in combination with cell culture for direct detection of respiratory viruses. J Clin Microbiol 1998;36:2112–4.
20. Weinberg A, Brewster L, Clark J, et al. Evaluation of R-Mix shell vials for the diagnosis of viral respiratory tract infections. J Clin Virol 2004;30:100–5.
21. Ladanyi A, Sher AC, Herlitz A, et al. Automated detection of immunofluorescently labeled cytomegalovirus-infected cells in isolated peripheral blood leukocytes using decision tree analysis. Cytometry A 2004;58:147–56.
22. Engvall E, Perlmann P. Enzyme-linked immunosorbent assay (ELISA). Quantitative assay of immunoglobulin G. Immunochemistry 1971;8:871–4.
23. Hornsleth A, Friis B, Andersen P, et al. Detection of respiratory syncytial virus in nasopharyngeal secretions by ELISA: comparison with fluorescent antibody technique. J Med Virol 1982;10:273–81.
24. McIntosh K, Hendry RM, Fahnestock ML, et al. Enzyme-linked immunosorbent assay for detection of respiratory syncytial virus infection: application to clinical samples. J Clin Microbiol 1982;16:329–33.
25. Harmon MW, Pawlik KM. Enzyme immunoassay for direct detection of influenza type A and adenovirus antigens in clinical specimens. J Clin Microbiol 1982;15:5–11.
26. Ohm-Smith MJ, Nassos PS, Haller BL. Evaluation of the Binax NOW, BD Directigen, and BD Directigen EZ assays for detection of respiratory syncytial virus. J Clin Microbiol 2004;42:2996–9.

27. Casiano-Colon AE, Hulbert BB, Mayer TK, et al. Lack of sensitivity of rapid antigen tests for the diagnosis of respiratory syncytial virus infection in adults. J Clin Virol 2003;28:169–74.
28. Hayden FG, Osterhaus AD, Treanor JJ, et al. Efficacy and safety of the neuraminidase inhibitor zanamivir in the treatment of influenzavirus infections. GG167 Influenza Study Group. N Engl J Med 1997;337:874–80.
29. Anonymous. Rapid diagnostic tests for influenza. Med Lett Drugs Ther 1999;41: 121–2.
30. Landry ML, Cohen S, Ferguson D. Comparison of Binax NOW and Directigen for rapid detection of influenza A and B. J Clin Virol 2004;31:113–5.
31. Zheng X, Quianzon S, Mu Y, et al. Comparison of two new rapid antigen detection assays for respiratory syncytial virus with another assay and shell vial culture. J Clin Virol 2004;31:130–3.
32. Ginocchio CC, Lotlikar M, Falk L, et al. Clinical performance of the 3M Rapid Detection Flu A+B Test compared to R-Mix culture, DFA and BinaxNOW Influenza A&B Test. J Clin Virol 2009;45:146–9.
33. Dale SE, Mayer C, Mayer MC, et al. Analytical and clinical sensitivity of the 3M rapid detection influenza A+B assay. J Clin Microbiol 2008;46:3804–7.
34. Newton DW, Mellen CF, Baxter BD, et al. Practical and sensitive screening strategy for detection of influenza virus. J Clin Microbiol 2002;40:4353–6.
35. Cruz AT, Cazacu AC, Greer JM, et al. Rapid assays for the diagnosis of influenza A and B viruses in patients evaluated at a large tertiary care children's hospital during two consecutive winter seasons. J Clin Virol 2008;41:143–7.
36. Hurt AC, Alexander R, Hibbert J, et al. Performance of six influenza rapid tests in detecting human influenza in clinical specimens. J Clin Virol 2007;39:132–5.
37. Nilsson AC, Alemo B, Bjorkman P, et al. Around-the-clock, rapid diagnosis of influenza by means of membrane chromatography antigen testing confirmed by polymerase chain reaction. Infect Control Hosp Epidemiol 2008;29:177–9.
38. Noyola DE, Clark B, O'Donnell FT, et al. Comparison of a new neuraminidase detection assay with an enzyme immunoassay, immunofluorescence, and culture for rapid detection of influenza A and B viruses in nasal wash specimens. J Clin Microbiol 2000;38:1161–5.
39. Mackie PL, McCormick EM, Williams C. Evaluation of Binax NOW RSV as an acute point-of-care screening test in a paediatric accident and emergency unit. Commun Dis Public Health 2004;7:328–30.
40. Shaw J, Vukajlovic S, Madse R, et al. Evaluation of the fluID™ rapid influenza test. In: 25th annual clinical virology symposium. Daytona Beach (FL); 2009.
41. Watanabe M, Nakagawa N, Ito M, et al. Sensitivity of rapid immunoassay for influenza A and B in the early phase of the disease. Pediatr Int 2009;51:211–5.
42. Chan KH, Peiris JS, Lim W, et al. Comparison of nasopharyngeal flocked swabs and aspirates for rapid diagnosis of respiratory viruses in children. J Clin Virol 2008;42:65–9.
43. Abu-Diab A, Azzeh M, Ghneim R, et al. Comparison between pernasal flocked swabs and nasopharyngeal aspirates for detection of common respiratory viruses in samples from children. J Clin Microbiol 2008;46:2414–7.

Antigen-Based Assays for the Identification of Influenza Virus and Respiratory Syncytial Virus: Why and How to Use Them in Pediatric Practice

Nicola Principi, MD*, Susanna Esposito, MD

KEYWORDS

- Influenza • Influenza virus • Respiratory syncytial virus
- Antigen-based assay • Pediatrics • Children

Respiratory tract infections are the most common diseases of infants and young children.[1–3] They are mainly caused by viruses, of which influenza viruses (IV) and respiratory syncytial virus (RSV) are the most important quantitatively and qualitatively.[4–6] Prompt identification of these viruses in the respiratory secretions of infected children is essential to plan adequate procedures to limit their spread, initiate antiviral therapy in patients at risk of complications, and avoid unnecessary drug prescriptions.[7,8]

Among the methods that have been developed to diagnose IV and RSV infections, serology cannot be used for a prompt diagnosis because it requires two blood samples, the second of which has to be drawn some weeks after the onset of symptoms.[9,10] Furthermore, cell cultures are complicated, expensive, and time consuming, and molecular assays have to be performed in particularly well equipped laboratories and cannot be used in an office or ambulatory care setting.[9,10] Antigen-based assays are inexpensive, easy to perform, and the result is available in a short time even in an ambulatory setting, or at least in some cases, at the patients' home.[9,10] For all these reasons, they are widely used in clinical practice.

This work was supported in part by a grant from the Italian Ministry of Universities, Project No. 2005068289_001.

Department of Maternal and Pediatric Sciences, University of Milan, Fondazione IRCCS Ospedale Maggiore Policlinico, Mangiagalli e Regina Elena, Via Commenda 9, 20122 Milano, Italy
* Corresponding author.
E-mail address: Nicola.Principi@unimi.it (N. Principi).

Clin Lab Med 29 (2009) 649–660
doi:10.1016/j.cll.2009.07.006
0272-2712/09/$ – see front matter © 2009 Elsevier Inc. All rights reserved.

The main aim of this article is to discuss the clinical and socioeconomic relevance of IV and RSV in pediatrics, the characteristics and limitations of the assays currently available, and the impact of rapid diagnostic tests.

EPIDEMIOLOGY AND CLINICAL PICTURE OF INFLUENZA VIRUSES AND RESPIRATORY SYNCYTIAL VIRUS INFECTIONS
Influenza Virus Infection

The use of reliable methods for identifying IV in the respiratory secretions of infants and children with fever or respiratory tract infection has made it possible to assess the importance of influenza in pediatrics. During every winter season, 10% to 30% of the pediatric population suffers from influenza, a significant number are hospitalized, and some even die.[7,11–13] The medical impact of pediatric influenza has been clearly demonstrated by Bourgeois and colleagues[12] in the United States, who estimated the number of patients younger than 7 years attending the emergency department of an urban tertiary care pediatric hospital with acute respiratory infection from 1993 to 2004 and found that 9.2% of all of the visits were associated with the detection of an IV in the respiratory secretions. Influenza led to the largest number of emergency department visits among children aged 6 to 23 months, but a significant number of visits (approximately 10%–12% for each age group) involved subjects aged 2 to 4 and 5 to 7 years.[12] Similar data have been collected by other authors in other countries; for example, we analyzed more than 3000 children with respiratory infection admitted to our emergency department in Italy during the influenza season of 2001 to 2002, and found that approximately 10% were suffering from laboratory-confirmed influenza.

After RSV, IV is the second most common respiratory virus causing hospitalization in children and adolescents. The incidence of hospitalization varies depending on the level of circulation of IV, the methods used to identify them, and the prevalence of high-risk children in the studied population. However, it is not less than 3.6 per 10,000 child-years, and is higher in younger children.[14,15] Finally, childhood influenza can be fatal. Given the high incidence of influenza infection, this event is fortunately rare but some dozens of influenza-associated deaths are recorded among pediatric patients every year in the United States.[13,16] Children with a chronic, severe underlying disease are at higher risk of complications when infected by IV than those uninfected, but contrary to what was supposed until the end of the last century, otherwise healthy patients can also suffer from severe influenza.[7,11–16] An evaluation of the 319 influenza-associated pediatric deaths reported in the United States from 2003 to 2007 has shown that approximately half had occurred in children without any risk factors.[16] This last finding can explain why the American Centers for Disease Control have recently suggested including all children aged 6 months to 18 years among those for whom influenza vaccination is recommended because of the high risk of influenza-related complications.[7] In addition, recent data show that hospitalization is common among children with an underlying chronic disease and those who are otherwise healthy. The studies published by Schrag and colleagues[14] and Coffin and colleagues[15] showed that, among 1308 and 745 hospitalized children with influenza respectively, 69% and approximately 50% did not have a medical condition associated with an increased risk of complications.

Influenza in children, with or without an underlying disease, is also a major economic problem because, in addition to the significant cost of medical visits and hospitalizations, it also increases the consumption of drugs, particularly antibiotics,[17–19] and has several indirect effects on the families of the infected children. Infected children are the most important cause of the spread of influenza because they shed more virus over a longer period than adults.[20] There are also data indicating that, in comparison with other respiratory viruses, IV have the highest negative impact on the family.[20–23] **Table 1** shows our findings demonstrating that the household contacts of a child with influenza require significantly more medical visits and miss significantly more working and school days during the week following the child's disease than those of children suffering from other respiratory viral infections.[23] Furthermore, even when not ill, parents can lose working days to stay at home to take care of their sick child or have to spend money to pay for help at home.[23] For all of these reasons, reducing the spread of influenza can be highly cost effective.

Influenza can be prevented by vaccination and antiviral drugs.[7] Unfortunately, influenza vaccines cannot be used in children aged less than 6 months and are not always effective, especially in younger patients. Moreover, although there is general agreement concerning their use in children with underlying chronic diseases, their administration to healthy patients is widely debated,[13] vaccination coverage remains generally low, and the risk of influenza in the pediatric population has not been significantly reduced by vaccine availability.[24] The prophylactic use of antivirals is only recommended in selected cases because, to be effective, these very expensive and not always well-tolerated drugs have to be administered every day for a long time.[7]

As in the case of RSV, an important way to reduce the circulation of IV is to identify infected children promptly, which is why rapid tests have been immediately adopted by hospitals and some primary care pediatricians.

Respiratory Syncytial Virus Infection

RSV is an RNA virus which, in temperate climates, is most active during the winter season.[4,5,25] It is the most important cause of pediatric respiratory tract infections because it infects almost all children in their first 2 years of life, and during this period, more than half the pediatric population suffers from at least two infections.[26] The severity of the respiratory tract involvement is mainly related to the age of the infected

Table 1
Social impact of influenza among the household contacts of otherwise healthy children with respiratory tract infections

	Household Contacts of Children with a Diagnosis of Influenza	
	Positive (n = 915)	Negative (n = 9,128)
Additional medical visits, mean ± SD	0.39 ± 0.76[a]	0.14 ± 0.47
Parents (%)	0.28 ± 0.55[a]	0.07 ± 0.25
Siblings (%)	0.48 ± 0.98[a]	0.22 ± 0.73
Lost working days (parents), mean ± SD	1.39 ± 3.09[a]	0.59 ± 2.02
Lost school days (siblings), mean ± SD	1.27 ± 2.47[a]	0.49 ± 2.33
Number of days on which help is needed to care for ill children, mean ± SD	1.10 ± 1.76[a]	0.85 ± 1.63

Abbreviation: SD, standard deviation.
[a] $P<.0001$ *versus* influenza-negative children; no other statistically significant differences.
Modified from Principi N, Esposito S, Marchisio P, et al. Socioeconomic impact of influenza in healthy children and their families. Pediatr Infect Dis J 2003;22:S207–10; with permission.[23]

child and the presence of an underlying chronic severe disease, including immunodeficiency caused by prematurity.[27]

RSV respiratory diseases are usually mild in healthy toddlers, older children, and adolescents because they mainly involve the upper respiratory tract or cause only transient wheezing.[28] However, during the first 2 years of life, most children with RSV infection manifest bronchiolitis whose particular clinical picture includes upper and lower respiratory tract involvement, respiratory distress, a harsh cough, bilateral crepitations, air trapping, and wheezing.[28] Although bronchiolitis has a self-limiting course in most children and can usually be managed conservatively at home, a number of cases require hospitalization because of marked hypoxia and the impossibility of maintaining adequate hydration and regular feeding.[8] It has been calculated that, every year, RSV causes 20,000 infant hospitalizations in the UK and 120,000 in the United States.[29,30] Approximately 1% of hospitalized children with bronchiolitis require admission to an intensive care unit (ICU), where mortality is less than 1% in otherwise healthy patients but can reach 3.5% in children at risk of cardiac or chronic lung disease.[8,29,30] These admission rates lead to high costs of care. Data collected in the United States show that RSV-associated morbidity during one season accounts for 13.5% to 21.6% of all charges attributable to lower-respiratory tract infections among hospitalized infants.[30]

Together with acute problems, children exposed to RSV infection in early life are at a higher risk of respiratory symptoms later on.[31–33] Approximately 50% of the infants hospitalized because of bronchiolitis experience subsequent episodes of wheezing, which, in some cases, may occur until they are 11 years old or older.[31–33] Among young school children, previous RSV infection may increase the risk of asthma 10 times.[31–33] The relationship between RSV infection during infancy and the future development of asthma is particularly clear in patients with a genetic predisposition for allergic diseases,[33] and recent data show that the number of RSV copies/mL and not the viral type at admission for bronchiolitis is significantly higher in children with recurrent wheezing than in those without (**Table 2**).[34]

RSV spreads readily in the community, particularly among children who have close contact with infected patients or contaminated surfaces or objects.[8,28] Nosocomial infections are common in pediatric wards.[35] Infection of adults living with infected children is less frequent, and so the social impact of RSV infection is less than that reported for influenza.[20]

However, the medical and economic impact of bronchiolitis explains why all of the measures theoretically capable of reducing the occurrence and spread of the infection have been widely studied, and when possible, implemented. Unfortunately, universal prevention is still not possible; there is no vaccine against RSV and the use of passive immunization has disadvantages, such that it can be suggested only for high-risk children.[8] Intravenous RSV immunoglobulins are very expensive, their administration requires a large fluid intake (with the risk of circulation problems), and their efficacy is poor because 17 infants have to be treated to prevent one hospitalization and 50 to prevent one ICU admission.[8] Humanized monoclonal antibodies are also expensive and reduce the hospitalization rate of children with bronchiolitis by no more than 50%.[36]

Consequently, the simplest and cheapest means of reducing the incidence of RSV disease is to limit the circulation of the virus and the risk of contagion. Together with the ways of preventing RSV transmission outlined by the American Academy of Pediatrics (frequent hand washing, the use and frequent changing of gloves, isolating or cohorting patients, and avoiding situations where exposure to RSV cannot be controlled), the prompt identification of infected children seems to be an important

Table 2
Relationship between respiratory syncytial virus and clinical data in children who have respiratory syncytial virus infection

Characteristic	RSV Viral Load (Copies/mL)	RSV A (n = 13) (%)	RSV B (n = 39) (%)
Rectal temperature			
≥38°C	$5.50 \times 10^5 \pm 2.01 \times 10^6$	3 (23.1)	11 (28.2)
<38°C	$4.20 \times 10^5 \pm 7.89 \times 10^5$	10 (76.9)	28 (71.8)
Severe symptoms			
Tachypnea ≥60 bpm.	$3.53 \times 10^5 \pm 8.17 \times 10^5$	8 (61.5)	22 (56.4)
Breath rate <60 bpm.	$6.59 \times 10^5 \pm 2.39 \times 10^6$	5 (38.5)	17 (43.6)
Pulse oximetry <92%	$7.06 \times 10^5 \pm 1.42 \times 10^6$	3 (23.1)	9 (23.1)
Pulse oximetry ≥92%	$4.75 \times 10^5 \pm 1.74 \times 10^6$	10 (76.9)	30 (76.9)
X ray			
Evidence of pneumonia	$6.03 \times 10^5 \pm 1.79 \times 10^6$	6 (46.2)	19 (48.7)
No evidence of pneumonia	$5.40 \times 10^5 \pm 2.10 \times 10^6$	7 (53.8)	20 (51.3)
Duration of hospitalization			
<4 d	$6.77 \times 10^5 \pm 2.40 \times 10^6$	6 (46.2)	19 (48.7)
≥4 d	$4.27 \times 10^5 \pm 9.98 \times 10^5$	7 (53.8)	20 (51.3)
Recurrent wheezing in the following 6 mo			
At least one episode of Wheezing	$8.27 \times 10^5 \pm 2.10 \times 10^{6a}$	8 (61.5)	24 (61.5)
No wheezing	$9.88 \times 10^2 \pm 2.41 \times 10^3$	5 (38.5)	15 (38.5)

Abbreviation: bpm, beats per minute.
[a] $P<.05$ *versus* no wheezing.
Modified from Bosis S, Esposito S, Niesters H, et al. Role of respiratory pathogens in infants hospitalized for their first episode of wheezing and their impact on subsequent recurrences. Clin Microbiol Infect 2008;14:677–84; with permission.[34]

means of reducing transmission.[10,37] A child infected by RSV can be isolated and all of the other measures can be implemented, which is why rapid tests for diagnosing RSV infection have been adopted by most hospitals and many primary care pediatricians.[10,37]

CHARACTERISTICS OF RAPID TESTS FOR INFLUENZA VIRUSES AND RESPIRATORY SYNCYTIAL VIRUS IDENTIFICATION
Rapid Influenza Tests

Several rapid influenza detection tests have been marketed. Most detect influenza A and B viruses, but only some can distinguish them.[38–40] The majority of the recently marketed tests are easy to use and do not require any particular laboratory experience. The specificity of these tests is typically greater than 90% and in many cases nearly 100%.[38,39] However, their sensitivity can vary from 10% to 96%,and in most cases, is approximately 60%,[38–40] which means that there is a high risk of false negative results, whereas the risk of false positives is low.

The variability in sensitivity is caused by many factors, including the standard used for comparison, the type of test, the circulating IV type/subtype, the type of specimen and when it is collected, and the patients' age.[38] Sensitivity is higher when rapid tests are compared with viral cultures rather than real-time polymerase chain reaction, because the latter is more sensitive for IV.[38] The importance of the type of kit was clearly demonstrated by the study of Hurt and colleagues,[40] who compared six rapid tests with cell cultures and found that five of them (Binax Now Influenza A&B, Directigen EZ Flu A + B, Denka Seiken Quick Ex-Flu, Fujirebio Espline Influenza A&B-N, and Quidel Quick Vue Influenza A + B Test) were 65% to 71% sensitive for influenza A, but one (Rockeby Influenza A Antigen Test) was only 10% sensitive. On the other hand, the same study showed that none of the tests with approximately 70% sensitivity for influenza A virus were more than 30% sensitive for influenza B.[40]

The role of specimen type has been evaluated in studies comparing nasopharyngeal (NP) aspirates and washes, posterior NP and throat swabs, sputum and bronchoalveolar lavage fluid.[41–43] Albeit with some exceptions,[41] nasal aspirates and washes were significantly superior to throat swabs.[42,43]

The higher level of viral shedding in infants and younger children is the main reason for the greater sensitivity of rapid influenza tests in patients aged less than 5 years.[44,45] Moreover, as viral shedding is greater during the first days of infection, sensitivity peaks in samples collected in the first 4 to 5 days after symptom onset.[44,45]

However, interpreting the results of even the most specific and sensitive tests depends on the prevalence of influenza in the community when the test is performed.[42,46–48] Grijalva and colleagues calculated the positive (PPV) and negative predictive value (NPV) of rapid tests with a mean sensitivity of 63% and a mean specificity of 97%, and found that PPV approached 80% when the prevalence of influenza was greater than or equal to 15%, but was no higher than 50% when it was 5%, whereas NPV was higher in the periods with the lowest circulation of IV and lower during epidemic peaks; when the prevalence of influenza was at its highest (60%) approximately 37% of the negative tests were false negatives.[42] However, it was calculated that a high risk of false negative tests was limited to periods when prevalence was more than 40%, a situation that is not common and does not last for more than a few days.[42]

All of these data clearly indicate that the real problem related to the use of rapid influenza tests is the risk of a false positive result when the prevalence of the infection is low. Outside the peak period, these tests do not offer any real advantage because approximately 50% of positive rapid tests could be false positives. This means that interpreting the results requires knowledge of the circulation of IV and the real prevalence of influenza infection.

Rapid Respiratory Syncytial Virus Tests

The antigen detection assays for diagnosing RSV infection include indirect and direct immunofluorescent antibody tests, enzyme immunoassays (EIA), and optical immunoassays.[10,49] Of those that are commercially available, EIA have the best combination of sensitivity, specificity, and ease of use, but as in the case of influenza detection assays, their specificity and (especially) sensitivity vary depending on the manufacturer, the virus and strain being detected, the age of the patients, and the adequacy of the specimen.[10,49] Moreover, in some cases, optimal sensitivity requires highly trained technologists and high-quality reagents and equipment; this is the case of direct immunofluorescence staining (DFA), which, although it has been reported to be the most sensitive rapid method of identifying RSV, is not used in many laboratories for these reasons.[50] Other tests, such as the Binax NOW RSV(BN) immunochromatographic assay (Binax, Inc, Portland, ME) and BD Directigen EZ RSV (BDEZ) immunochromatographic assay (Becton Dickinson and Company, Sparks, MD) have rapid processing times and require, at most, only one preparation step.[51] Therefore, these tests can be used at the bedside or in an outpatient setting, even by a variety of medical personnel.

Generally speaking, the same conclusions as those reported for IV detection tests apply to rapid RSV tests. Most of the tests have a specificity of more than 90%, but their sensitivity is less and can vary from test to test even when evaluating the same sample.[10,49–56] Ohm-Smith and colleagues[50] compared four rapid RSV assays with cultures, and found that the specificity of DFA, BN, BD Directigen, and BDEZ were practically equivalent (always higher than 96%), but their sensitivity was significantly different (93%, 89%, 59%, and 77%, respectively) (**Table 3**). When the results were divided into those of children and adults, DFA was the only adequate test for detecting RSV in adults: 100% sensitivity, compared with 0% for BN, 0% for BD Directigen, and 25% for BDEZ.[50] On the contrary, the differences were significantly less evident in children: 93% for DFA, 94% for BN, 72% for BD Directigen, and 81% for BDEZ.[50] Similar data showing that all of the rapid RSV detection tests are more reliable in children have been reported by other authors.[52–54] This confirms what has previously been demonstrated in the case of IV assays, and can once again be ascribed to the higher concentrations of infectious agents in samples collected from younger subjects. However, Selvarangan and colleagues[55] found significantly better BDEZ data in a pediatric population, and demonstrated the substantial equivalence of BN (specificity and sensitivity: 100% and 90%) and BDEZ (94% and 90%). It remains to be clarified whether RSV detection is better in nasal aspirates or washes than in nasal swabs.[49–56]

As previously discussed for IV antigen assays, the reliability of the results of RSV strictly depends on the prevalence of the virus in the community, and is low outside the peak period, when the risk of false positives can be so high that the use of the tests seems debatable.[57,58]

IMPACT OF RAPID TESTS FOR INFLUENZA VIRUSES AND RESPIRATORY SYNCYTIAL INFECTIONS ON CLINICAL PEDIATRIC PRACTICE

Although rapid tests for the identification of IV and RSV antigens have been mainly developed to allow the prompt implementation of methods useful for reducing the spread of the viruses, their use in clinical practice can led to a number of other positive results.[59]

This claim is particularly true of rapid IV tests, as most of the data concerning their use in children with respiratory infections or sourceless fever indicate that they decrease: (1) the need for an additional diagnostic work-up, including complete blood counts, blood cultures, urinalyses, urine cultures, and chest radiographs; (2) the costs

Table 3
Evaluation of rapid assays for the detection of respiratory syncytial virus in comparison with culture

Test	Sensitivity (%)	Specificity (%)	Positive Predictive Value (%)	Negative Predictive Value (%)
DFA	93	97	93	97
DRSV	77	96	88	92
NOW	89	100	100	95
BD Directigen EZ	59	98	93	88

Abbreviations: DRSV, BD Directigen RSV enzyme immunoassay (Becton Dickinson and Company, Sparks, MD).

Modified from Ohm-Smith MJ, Nassos PS, Haller BL. Evaluation of the Binax NOW, BD Directigen, and BD Directigen EZ assays for detection of respiratory syncytial virus. *Data from* J Clin Microbiol 2004;42:2996–9.[50]

associated with these tests; and (3) the number of prescribed antibiotic courses.[60–62] Further benefits shown by some studies are a reduced length of stay in the emergency department and a reduced likelihood of hospital admission.[60,62] Moreover, the more appropriate use of antivirals, such as oseltamivir and zanamivir, has been demonstrated in the case of a positive diagnosis.[62]

The benefits associated with rapid tests were clear in a study by our group that compared pediatricians' behavior when the patients had a negative test, a positive test, or the absence of any result.[61] We found that pediatricians behaved in the same way when a test is negative or not done at all, because in both cases, they prescribed significantly more ancillary tests and antibiotic courses than when they knew the child really has influenza (**Table 4**). The reduced number of ancillary tests has mainly economic value, but the decrease in antibiotic use can also have significant medical consequences because it reduces drug-related adverse events and limits the risk of the emergence of antibiotic resistant bacteria, which, in an age of increasing antibiotic resistance, is an advantage that should not be underestimated.

Table 4
Comparison of children with a positive or negative rapid influenza test result

Characteristic	Cases (n = 43) (%)	Control Group 1 (n = 435) (%)	P Value	Control Group 2 (n = 479) (%)	P Value
Gender					
Male	23 (53.5)	242 (55.6)	0.913	254 (53.0)	0.919
Female	20 (46.5)	193 (44.4)	—	225 (47.0)	—
Age (y)					
Median	2.5	2.3	0.643	2.6	0.706
Range	0.3–14.5	0.1–14.7	—	0.1–14.8	—
Previous influenza vaccination	0	9 (2.1)	1.000	11 (2.3)	0.611
Diagnosis					
Rhinitis	14 (32.6)	105 (24.1)	0.301	137 (28.6)	0.709
Pharyngitis	16 (37.2)	163 (37.5)	0.133	164 (34.2)	0.821
Acute otitis media	9 (20.9)	72 (16.6)	0.605	86 (18.0)	0.725
Croup	1 (2.3)	8 (1.8)	0.575	15 (3.1)	1.000
Wheezing	1 (2.3)	20 (4.6)	0.709	19 (4.0)	1.000
Acute bronchitis	2 (4.7)	41 (9.4)	0.408	34 (7.1)	0.757
Pneumonia	0	26 (6.0)	0.153	24 (5.0)	0.246
Routine blood examination	1 (2.3)	63 (14.5)	0.045	72 (15.0)	0.038
Chest radiograph	2 (4.6)	50 (11.5)	0.207	56 (11.7)	0.208
Antibiotic use	14 (32.6)	282 (64.8)	<0.0001	296 (61.8)	0.0003
Days of antibiotics					
Median	7	7	0.944	7	0.961
Range	4–10	3–20	—	5–14	—
Admitted	0	20 (4.6)	0.240	28 (5.8)	0.154

Control group 1 refers to children with a positive (cases) or negative rapid influenza test result and control group 2 refers to those who did not undergo the test.

Modified from Esposito S, Marchisio P, Morelli P, et al. Effect of a rapid influenza test. *Data from* Arch Dis Child 2003;88:525–6.[61]

Finally, a particular advantage of using rapid influenza tests is the possibility of avoiding blood cultures to diagnose serious bacterial infections (SBI) in younger children with sourceless fever and positive IV detection. Smitherman and colleagues[63] compared the incidence of SBI in infants aged 0 to36 months with fever and influenza A infection with that in subjects without influenza, and found that the risk of SBI was significantly lower in the former.

Similar data have been collected regarding the impact of RSV detection tests in clinical practice, particularly the reduction in antibiotic use.[64] Moreover, because the risk of SBI is significantly lower in RSV-infected children aged less than 2 months of age than in those without RSV infection, the use of rapid tests can eliminate the need for blood cultures.[57,58]

SUMMARY

Rapid tests for the identification of IV and RSV in the respiratory secretions of infants and children are useful in improving the diagnosis of common and possibly severe diseases, such as influenza and bronchiolitis. Their sensitivity and specificity mean that they are most reliable when the prevalence of infection is high, which suggests that their routine use should be limited to the peak periods of viral circulation. As the most recently marketed tests are similarly effective in identifying the viruses, pediatricians should choose those that are less expensive, less time consuming, and easier to perform and interpret.

REFERENCES

1. Feigin RD, Cherry JD, editors. Textbook of pediatric infectious diseases. 4th edition. Philadelphia: W.B. Saunders Company; 1998.
2. Principi N, Esposito S. Emerging role of Mycoplasma pneumoniae and Chlamydia pneumoniae in paediatric respiratory tract infections. Lancet Infect Dis 2001;1: 334–44.
3. Ramsey CD, Gold DR, Litonjua AA, et al. Respiratory illnesses in early life and asthma and atopy in childhood. J Allergy Clin Immunol 2007;119:150–6.
4. Esposito S, Gasparini R, Bosis S, et al. Clinical and socioeconomic impact of influenza and respiratory syncytial virus (RSV) infection on healthy children and their households. Clin Microbiol Infect 2005;11:933–6.
5. Gasparini R, Durando P, Ansaldi F, et al. Influenza and respiratory syncytial virus in infants and children: relationship with attendance at a paediatric emergency unit and characteristics of the circulating strains. Eur J Clin Microbiol Infect Dis 2007;26:619–28.
6. Bosis S, Esposito S, Niesters HGM, et al. Impact of human metapneumovirus in childhood: comparison with respiratory syncytial virus and influenza viruses. J Med Virol 2005;75:101–4.
7. Centers for Disease Control and Prevention (CDC). Prevention and control of influenza. Recommendations of the Advisory Committee on Immunization Practices (ACIP). MMWR Morb Mortal Wkly Rep 2008;57(RR07):1–59.
8. American Academy of Pediatrics. Subcommittee on Diagnosis and Management of Bronchiolitis. Diagnosis and management of bronchiolitis. Pediatrics 2006;118: 1774–93.
9. Glezen WP. Modifying clinical practices to manage influenza in children effectively. Pediatr Infect Dis J 2008;27:738–43.
10. Henrickson KJ, Breese Hall C. Diagnostic assays for respiratory syncytial virus disease. Pediatr Infect Dis J 2007;26:S36–40.

11. Bhat N, Wright JG, Broder KR, et al. Influenza associated deaths among children in the United States, 2003–2004. N Engl J Med 2005;353:2559–67.
12. Bourgeois FT, Valim C, Wei JC, et al. Influenza and other respiratory virus-related emergency department visits among young children. Pediatrics 2006; 118:e1–8.
13. Esposito S, Marchisio P, Principi N. The global state of influenza in children. Pediatr Infect Dis J 2008;27(Suppl 11):s149–53.
14. Schrag SJ, Shay DK, Gershman K, et al. Multistate surveillance for laboratory-confirmed, influenza-associated hospitalizations in children: 2003–2004. Pediatr Infect Dis J 2006;25:395–400.
15. Coffin SE, Zaoutis TE, Rosenquist AB, et al. Incidence, complications, and risk factors for prolonged stay in children hospitalized with community-acquired influenza. Pediatrics 2007;119:740–8.
16. Finelli L, Fiore A, Dhara R, et al. Influenza-associated pediatric mortality in the United States: increase of Staphylococcus aureus coinfection. Pediatrics 2008; 122:805–11.
17. Principi N, Esposito S. Are we ready for universal influenza vaccination in paediatrics? Lancet Infect Dis 2004;4:75–83.
18. Poehling KA, Edwards KM, Weinberg GA, et al. The under-recognized burden of influenza in young children. N Engl J Med 2006;355:31–40.
19. Neuzil KM, Hohlbein C, Zhu Y. Illness among schoolchildren during influenza season. Effect on school absenteeism, parental absenteeism from work, and secondary illness in families. Arch Pediatr Adolesc Med 2002; 156:986–91.
20. Principi N, Esposito S, Bosis S. Human metapneumovirus and lower respiratory tract disease in children. N Engl J Med 2004;350:1788–90.
21. Esposito S, Bosis S, Niesters HG, et al. Impact of human bocavirus on children and their families. J Clin Microbiol 2008;46:1337–42.
22. Principi N, Esposito S. Prevention or control of influenza in the pediatric population. Emerg Infect Dis 2004;10:574–80.
23. Principi N, Esposito S, Marchisio P, et al. Socioeconomic impact of influenza in healthy children and their families. Pediatr Infect Dis J 2003;22:s207–10.
24. Esposito S, Marchisio P, Droghetti R, et al. Influenza vaccination coverage among children with high-risk medical conditions. Vaccine 2006;24:5251–5.
25. DeVincenzo JP. Natural infection of infants with respiratory syncytial virus subgroups A and B: a study of frequency, disease severity, and viral load. Pediatr Res 2004;56:914–7.
26. Somech R, Tal G, Gilad E, et al. Epidemiologic, socioeconomic, and clinical factors associated with severity of respiratory syncytial virus infection in previously healthy infants. Clin Pediatr 2006;45:621–7.
27. Rossi GA, Medici MC, Arcangeletti MC, et al. Risk factors for severe RSV-induced lower respiratory tract infection over four consecutive epidemics. Eur J Pediatr 2007;166:1267–72.
28. Nokes JD, Cane PA. New strategies for control of respiratory syncytial virus infection. Curr Opin Infect Dis 2008;21:639–43.
29. Sikkel MB, Quint JK, Mallia P, et al. Respiratory syncytial virus persistence in chronic obstructive pulmonary disease. Pediatr Infect Dis J 2008;27(Suppl 10): S63–70.
30. Stang P, Brandeburg N, Carter B. The economic burden of respiratory syncytial virus-associated bronchiolitis hospitalizations. Arch Pediatr Adolesc Med 2001; 155:95–6.

31. Sigurs N, Bjamason R, Sigurbergsson F, et al. Respiratory syncytial virus bronchiolitis in infancy is an important risk factor for asthma and allergy at age 7. Am J Respir Crit Care Med 2000;161:1501–7.
32. Stein RT, Sherill D, Morgan WJ, et al. Respiratory syncytial virus in early life and risk of wheeze and allergy by age 13 years. Lancet 1999;354:541–5.
33. Singh AM, Moore PE, Gern JE, et al. Bronchiolitis to asthma: a review and call for studies of gene-virus interactions in asthma causation. Am J Respir Crit Care Med 2007;175:108–19.
34. Bosis S, Esposito S, Niesters H, et al. Role of respiratory pathogens in infants hospitalized for their first episode of wheezing and their impact on subsequent recurrences. Clin Microbiol Infect 2008;14:677–84.
35. Groothuis J, Bauman J, Malinoski F, et al. Strategies for prevention of RSV nosocomial infection. J Perinatol 2008;28:319–23.
36. Simoes EA, Groothuis JR, Carbonell-Estrany X, et al. Palivizumab prophylaxis, respiratory syncytial virus, and subsequent recurrent wheezing. J Pediatr 2007; 151:34–42.
37. Greenough A. Respiratory syncytial virus infection: clinical features, management, and prophylaxis. Curr Opin Pulm Med 2002;8:214–7.
38. Uyeki T. Influenza diagnosis and treatment in children: a review of studies on clinically useful tests and antiviral treatment for influenza. Pediatr Infect Dis J 2003;22:164–77.
39. Grijalva CG, Poehling KA, Edwarda KM, et al. Accuracy and interpretation of rapid influenza tests in children. Pediatrics 2007;119:e6–11.
40. Hurt AC, Alexander R, Hibbert J, et al. Performance of six influenza rapid tests in detecting human influenza in clinical specimens. J Clin Virol 2007;39:132–5.
41. Covalciuc KA, Webb KH, Carlson CA. Comparison of four clinical specimen types for detection of influenza A and B viruses by optical immunoassay (FLU OIA test) and cell culture methods. J Clin Microbiol 1999;37:3971–4.
42. Heikkinen T, Marttila J, Salmi AA, et al. Nasal swab versus nasopharyngeal aspirate for isolation of respiratory viruses. J Clin Microbiol 2002;40:4337–9.
43. Lambert SB, Whiley DM, O'Neill NT, et al. Comparing nose-throat swabs and nasopharyngeal aspirates collected from children with symptoms for respiratory virus identification using real-time polymerase chain reaction. Pediatrics 2008; 122:e615–20.
44. Benito-Fernandez J, Vasquez-Ronco MA, Morteruel-Aizkuren E, et al. Impact of rapid viral testing for influenza A and B viruses on management of febrile infants without signs of focal infection. Pediatr Infect Dis J 2006;25:1153–7.
45. Pierron S, Haas H, Berlioz M, et al. Impact of rapid influenza test during influenza epidemic in all febrile children less than 6 years old in a pediatric emergency department. Arch Pediatr 2008;15:1283–8.
46. Weinberg A, Walker ML. Evaluation of three immunoassay kits for rapid detection of influenza virus A and B. Clin Diagn Lab Immunol 2005;12:367–70.
47. Agoritsas K, Mack K, Bonsu BK, et al. Evaluation of the Quidel QuickVue test for detection of influenza A and B viruses in the pediatric emergency medicine setting by use of three specimen collection methods. J Clin Microbiol 2006;44:2638–41.
48. Cruz AT, Cazacu AC, Greer JM, et al. Rapid assays for the diagnosis of influenza A and B viruses in patients evaluated at a large tertiary care children's hospital during two consecutive winter seasons. J Clin Virol 2008;41:143–7.
49. Aslanzadeh J, Zheng X, Li H, et al. Prospective evaluation of rapid antigen tests for diagnosis of respiratory syncytial virus and human metapneumovirus infections. J Clin Microbiol 2008;46:1682–5.

50. Ohm-Smith MJ, Nassos PS, Haller BL. Evaluation of the Binax NOW, BD Directigen, and BD Directigen EZ assays for detection of respiratory syncytial virus. J Clin Microbiol 2004;42:2996–9.
51. Liao RS, Tomalty LL, Majury A, et al. A comparison of viral isolation and multiplex real-time reverse transcription-PCR for the confirmation of respiratory syncytial virus and influenza viruses detected by antigen immunoassay. J Clin Microbiol 2009;47:527–32.
52. Reina J, Gonzalez GM, Ruiz DG, et al. Prospective evaluation of a dot-blot enzyme immunoassay (Directigen RSV) for the antigen detection of respiratory syncytial virus from nasopharyngeal aspirates of paediatric patients. Clin Microbiol Infect 2004;10:967–71.
53. Slinger R, Milk R, Gaboury I, et al. Evaluation of the QuickLab RSV test, a new rapid lateral-flow immunoassay for detection of respiratory syncytial virus antigen. J Clin Microbiol 2004;42:3731–3.
54. Zheng X, Quianzon S, Mu Y, et al. Comparison of two new rapid antigen detection assays for respiratory syncytial virus with another assay and shell vial culture. J Clin Virol 2004;31:130–3.
55. Selvarangan R, Abel D, Hamilton M. Comparison of BD Directigen™ EZ RSV and Binax NOW RSV tests for rapid detection of respiratory syncytial virus from nasopharyngeal aspirates in a pediatric population. Diagn Microbiol Infect Dis 2008; 62:157–61.
56. Schützle H, Weigl J, Puppe W, et al. Diagnostic performance of a rapid antigen test for RSV in comparison with a 19-valent multiplex RT-PCR ELISA in children with acute respiratory tract infections. Eur J Pediatr 2008;167:745–9.
57. Titus MO, Wright SW. prevalence of serious bacterial infections in febrile infants with respiratory syncytial virus infection. Pediatrics 2003;112:282–4.
58. Levine DA, Platt SL, Dayan PS, et al. Risk of serious bacterial infection in young febrile infants with respiratory syncytial virus infection. Pediatrics 2004;113: 1728–34.
59. Vega R. Rapid viral testing in the evaluation of the febrile infant and child. Curr Opin Pediatr 2005;17:363–7.
60. Sharma V, Dowd MD, Slaughter AJ, et al. Effect of rapid diagnosis of influenza virus type A on the emergency department management of febrile infants and toddlers. Arch Pediatr Adolesc Med. 2002;156:41–3.
61. Esposito S, Marchisio P, Morelli P, et al. Effect of a rapid influenza test. Arch Dis Child 2003;88:525–6.
62. Bonner AB, Monroe KW, Talley LI, et al. Impact of the rapid diagnosis of influenza on physician decision-making and patient management in the pediatric emergency department: results of a randomized, prospective, controlled trial. Pediatrics 2003;112:363–7.
63. Smitherman HF, Caviness AC, Macias CG. Retrospective review of serious bacterial infections in infants who are 0 to 36 months and have influenza A infection. Pediatrics 2005;115:710–9.
64. Byington CL, Castillo H, Gerber K, et al. The effect of rapid respiratory viral diagnostic testing on antibiotic use in a children's hospital. Arch Pediatr Adolesc Med 2002;156:1230–4.

Utilization of Nucleic Acid Amplification Assays for the Detection of Respiratory Viruses

Sue C. Kehl, PhD[a,b,*], Swati Kumar, MD[b,c]

KEYWORDS

- Nucleic acid amplification assays • Respiratory virus
- Influenza • Respiratory syncytial virus
- Molecular methods • PCR

Viruses are major contributors to morbidity and mortality from acute respiratory infections (ARIs) in all age groups worldwide. In addition to the enormous burden of upper respiratory syndromes caused by them, they are a leading cause of hospitalizations for lower respiratory infections (LRIs) in all age groups. Estimates of the national disease burden of respiratory viruses report that approximately 300,000 children are hospitalized each year in the United States with a specific diagnosis of viral LRI, and an additional 500,000 children are hospitalized with a clinical diagnosis of viral LRI, at a direct cost estimated at nearly $1 billion per year.[1] Rapid viral diagnosis has been demonstrated to significantly decrease length of hospital stay, additional laboratory testing, and unnecessary antibiotic use; it additionally helps direct specific antiviral therapy.[2,3]

Accurate identification of the etiologic agent of respiratory tract infections is important for proper patient management. Diagnosis can be problematic, because a range of potential pathogens can cause similar clinical symptoms. Nucleic acid amplification testing is emerging as the preferred method of diagnostic testing. Real-time technology and the ability to perform multiplex testing have facilitated this emergence. Commercial methodologies for nucleic acid amplification testing of respiratory viruses

[a] Department of Pathology, Medical College of Wisconsin, 9200 W. Wisconsin Avenue, PO Box 26509, Milwaukee, WI 53226-0509, USA
[b] Microbiology, Children's Hospital of Wisconsin, 9000 W. Wisconsin Avenue, PO Box 1997, Milwaukee, WI 53201-1997, USA
[c] Division of Infectious Diseases, Medical College of Wisconsin, 999 N. 92nd street Suite C450, PO Box 26509, Milwaukee, WI 53226-0509, USA
* Corresponding author. Department of Pathology, Medical College of Wisconsin, Post Office Box 26509, Milwaukee, WI 53226-0509.
E-mail address: kskehl@mcw.edu (S.C. Kehl).

Clin Lab Med 29 (2009) 661–671
doi:10.1016/j.cll.2009.07.008
0272-2712/09/$ – see front matter © 2009 Elsevier Inc. All rights reserved.

labmed.theclinics.com

include real-time polymerase chain reaction (PCR), nucleic acid sequence-based amplification (NASBA), and loop-mediated isothermal amplification (LAMP). Multiplex PCR with fluidic microarrays or DNA chips is the most recent diagnostic advance. Before the issuance of the guidance document on analyte-specific reagents (ASRs) by the US Food and Drug Administration (FDA),[4] primers and probes were being developed, packaged, and sold as ASRs. Since then, some of these reagents are no longer commercially available; some have been submitted and received FDA approval as in vitro diagnostic devices, and some primer and probe reagents are sold separately without recommendations for use. This article discusses commercially available molecular methods and their performance characteristics for the detection of respiratory viruses.

COMMERCIALLY AVAILABLE ASSAYS FOR THE DETECTION OF RESPIRATORY VIRUSES
Influenza Virus

Influenza viruses remain significant causes of ARI every year despite availability of vaccines and increasing efforts to achieve targeted vaccination rates. In 1998, these viruses were estimated to cause 39,000 hospitalizations per year in children nationally in the US.[1] The outpatient visits associated with influenza were reported to be approximately 10, 100, and 250 times as high as hospitalization rates for children 0 to 5 months, 6 to 23 months, and 24 to 59 months of age, respectively.[5] Substantial burden from influenza-associated hospitalizations and deaths has been ascertained in several studies, most severely affecting those older than 65 years but also being significant in the 50- to 65-year-old adults, in whom hospitalization rates were determined to equal those among children younger than 5 years.[6] Antigen assays for the detection of influenza are commonly available. The likelihood of a negative result using these assays increases significantly with the increasing age of the patient, whereas virus culture and reverse transcriptase PCR (RT-PCR) do not; for older patients, RT-PCR or culture is necessary to avoid false-negative results.[7]

Molecular methods for detecting influenza viruses were described as early as 1991. Various targets, including the matrix, HA, and N genes have been used. The first commercially available assay was the Hexaplex assay (Prodesse Inc, Waukesha, Wisconsin), an RT-PCR assay that employed enzyme hybridization postamplification detection. The assay was technically demanding, requiring postamplification purification; it was also expensive and took 8 to 9 hours to complete.[8] This assay had an analytical sensitivity of 10 copies for influenza A and 5 copies for influenza B[9] and set the standard for the detection of influenza viruses. Since then, it has been redesigned and is now an FDA-approved multiplex real-time RT-PCR assay (Pro-Flu+, Prodesse Inc,) for detecting influenza A (M gene), influenza B (NS1 and NS2 genes), and respiratory syncytial virus (RSV) (polymerase gene). It can be performed using a MagNA Pure LC Instrument (Roche Diagnostics Corporation, Indianapolis, Indiana), or the NucliSens easyMAG System (bioMerieux Inc, Durham, North Carolina) for extraction with amplification and detection on the SmartCycler system (Cepheid, Sunnyvale, California). According to the manufacturer, it has a clinical sensitivity and specificity of 100% and 93% for influenza A and 98% and 99% for influenza B, respectively, and an analytical sensitivity of 10^2 50% tissue culture infectious dose ($TCID_{50}$)/mL for both viruses. The xTAG Respiratory Virus Panel (Luminex Molecular Diagnostics, Toronto, Canada) also is an FDA-approved multiplex panel for detecting respiratory viruses. While capable of detecting 17 respiratory viruses, it is FDA-approved for detecting RSV; parainfluenza 1, 2, and 3; metapneumovirus; adenovirus, and rhinovirus, in addition to influenza. The assay employs multiplex PCR and fluid microsphere-based array detection on the Luminex x-MAP system (flow cytometer). It has a reported clinical sensitivity of 100% for influenza A[10] and an analytical sensitivity of 10 $TCID_{50}$.[11] In addition to these FDA-approved assays, ASRs for influenza are commercially available from EraGen Biosciences (Madison, Wisconsin) and Cepheid (Sunnyvale, California). These assays have no performance claims made by the manufacturer, and little information is published regarding their performance. The literature is replete with home-brew or in-house developed assays for detecting influenza using various amplification methodologies. In evaluating a home-brew assay or an ASR, an analytical sensitivity of 10 $TCID_{50}$ is desirable. In comparison with antigen assays and culture, clinical sensitivity of 98% to 99% should be easily attainable, along with the detection of additional viruses missed by culture. An alternate PCR methodology can confirm these as true positive specimens. PCR-based respiratory virus assays have demonstrated significantly better sensitivity than antigen detection assays, both enzyme immunoassays[7,12] where adults may have a false-negative rate of up to 29%,[13] and immunofluorescent assays[14] They also have better sensitivity than culture[15,16] in children[17] and particularly in adults.[18-20] Several manufacturers have assays available as research use only (RUO) kits. There are several kits, the Multi-Code-PLx (EraGen Biosciences, Inc) and the ResPlex II Panel (Qiagen Inc, Valencia, California), that employ the Luminex system, and these have reported performance claims similar to the xTAG Respiratory Virus Panel.[21,22,23] Automated solid film microarray assays also are being developed,[24] but none are commercially available.

Respiratory Syncytial Virus

Respiratory syncytial virus (RSV) is accepted as the most important respiratory viral pathogen in infants and young children. It long has been recognized to cause the highest number of pediatric hospitalizations from LRI, with estimates of more than 90,000 to 112,000 hospitalizations annually in children younger than 5 years.[1] Subsequent studies have shed light on the enormous outpatient and emergency room burden of illness associated with this virus also.[25] Thus, in addition to causing annual winter epidemics of bronchiolitis and pneumonia in young children requiring hospitalization, RSV also leads to significant outpatient disease. The virus further has been established as an important pathogen of respiratory disease in the elderly and high-risk adults.[26]

Like influenza, the Hexaplex assay was the first commercially available assay for detecting RSV. It had an analytical sensitivity of 42 to 4200 copies[8] and a clinical sensitivity and specificity of 99% and 97%, respectively, in children[12] and 91% and 99% in a mixed population of adults and children.[8] It, too, has been redesigned into the FDA-approved multiplex real-time RT-PCR assay, the Pro-Flu+, which, according to the manufacturer, has an analytical sensitivity of 10^{-1} to 10^{1} $TCID_{50}$ and a clinical sensitivity and specificity of 90% and 95%, respectively. In a study of an earlier version performed on pediatric samples, the assay had a sensitivity and specificity of 99% and 100%.[17] The assay has a sensitivity of 95% as compared with 82% for the enzyme immunoassay and 57% for culture.[27] The FDA-approved xTAG Respiratory Virus Panel has an analytical sensitivity of 10^{2} $TCID_{50}$/reaction[11] and a clinical sensitivity of 97%. The ASR commercially available from Cepheid has an analytical sensitivity of 12 copies per reaction and a clinical sensitivity of 100% when compared with enzyme immunoassay. A 22% increase in positive patients, however, was seen with the ASR. This increased positivity rate by RT-PCR is consistent with that reported by others when compared with antigen detection methods.[28] In-house assays for detecting RSV have been developed using the F, N, or L polymerase gene targets. These studies report 82% sensitivity of the antigen assay,[29] low sensitivity of culture,[30] and an increase in detection of positive patients by RT-PCR.[14,31] This increased sensitivity of RT-PCR has been reported in immunocompromised adults also.[32] Nucleic acid amplification assays are the most sensitive method for the detection of RSV[30] regardless of the population tested. Specimens with low viral load, as is seen in adults and immunocompromised patients, are more likely to be antigen-negative and RT-PCR positive[14,27] The MultiCode-PLx RUO assay has reported performance claims similar to the xTAG Respiratory Virus Panel,[21,34] while the ResPlex II Panel RUO assay has a significantly lower sensitivity of 73%.[22] Automated microarrays are being developed for RSV also.[24]

Parainfluenza

Human parainfluenzaviruses types 1, 2, and 3 (HPIV-1, HPIV-2, and HPIV-3) are important causes of ARI in all age groups. They cause upper respiratory tract infections (croup) in both children and adults, and lower respiratory tract infections in infants, young children, the elderly, the immunocompromised, or those with chronic medical conditions.[35] HPIVs are second only to RSV as a cause of hospitalizations for LRI in children[1,35] The different subtypes are associated with distinct clinical syndromes, age groups, and seasonality.[35] The clinical significance and epidemiology of a fourth type (HPIV-4), although discovered more than 40 years ago, are understood less well than the other three types.

The only FDA-approved assay for detecting HPIV-1, 2, and 3 is the xTAG Respiratory Virus Panel. It has an analytical sensitivity 100, 100, and 25 $TCID_{50}$/reaction[11] and a clinical sensitivity of 100%, 92% and 100% for HPIV-1, 2, and 3, respectively[10] The MultiCode-PLx RUO assay has reported sensitivity of 85% to 90%,[34,23] while the ResPlex II Panel RUO assay has a significantly lower sensitivity of 72% for HPIV-3.[22] These evaluations suffer from a low number of positive samples, particularly for HPIV-2. The Pro-Paraflu+ assay from Prodesse is also an RUO assay; however, there are no published reports of its performance. The Hexaplex assay had reported sensitivity of 100% for parainfluenzaviruses with an increased detection in the number of positive patients, suggesting that it was more sensitive than culture[8,12] and that sensitivity of this nature is achievable with the proper primers, probes, and conditions. Other in-house developed assays have reported similar findings.[14,36] A study comparing an in-house assay with direct fluorescent antigen reported a sensitivity of only 52% for antigen detection and 99% for RT-PCR.[14] Nucleic acid amplification assays are preferable to direct fluorescent antigen assays and culture for detecting parainfluenzaviruses.

Adenovirus

Adenoviruses are ubiquitously distributed viruses that are common causes of self-limiting respiratory, ocular, or gastrointestinal illnesses and outbreaks in immunocompetent children and United States military recruits. They have been reported to cause severe, prolonged, and sometimes fatal illness in immunocompromised hosts. The spectrum of disease in the latter population includes pneumonia, hepatitis, hemorrhagic cystitis, colitis, pancreatitis, myocarditis, meningoencephalitis, and disseminated disease, depending on host and virus characteristics.[37] Seven species (A to G) and 52 serotypes have been described, some associated with distinct clinical syndromes involving specific organ systems.

Most nucleic acid amplification assays for detecting adenovirus detect the hexon gene although assays targeting the fiber gene have been reported. The xTAG Respiratory Virus Panel is the only FDA-approved assay for detecting adenovirus from respiratory specimens. It has an analytical sensitivity of 10^2 $TCID_{50}$/reaction and a clinical sensitivity of 78%.[33] Adenovirus also is included in the MultiCode-PLx RUO assay and has reported sensitivity of 100%; however, only a small number of positive samples were tested.[21] An in-house developed assay targeting the hexon gene has a clinical sensitivity of 98%, with indirect immunofluorescent antigen test having a sensitivity of only 24%. This study also showed a several log difference in the concentration of viruses in specimens positive by PCR alone as compared with specimens positive by both immunofluorescent antigen testing and PCR.[14] Well-designed nucleic acid amplification assays that can detect all of the adenovirus serotypes are the most sensitive method for the detection of adenovirus. Because of the wide spectrum of disease, validation of the assay with a wide range of specimen types is important.

Metapneumovirus

Human metapneumovirus (hMPV), the most well-studied of the new viruses, was discovered in 2001; since then, it has been established as a significant respiratory pathogen in children and adults.[38,39] It has been reported to be the second most common causative agent in bronchiolitis in infants, and it contributes to a substantial burden of upper respiratory tract infections including acute otitis media in older children. The virus is a common cause of mild upper respiratory infection (URI) or asymptomatic illness in healthy adults. Severe illness resulting in hospitalizations including ICU admissions has been described in the elderly, adults with underlying conditions, and the immunocompromised.[39]

The xTAG Respiratory Virus Panel is an FD- approved assay for detecting hMPV from respiratory specimens. It has an analytical sensitivity of 0.1 $TCID_{50}$/mL and a clinical sensitivity of 97%,[33] detecting significantly more positives than the direct immunofluorescent assay. Pro-hMPV+ (Prodesse) is an FDA-approved real-time RT-PCR. According to the manufacturer, it has an analytical sensitivity of 10^1 to 10^2 $TCID_{50}$ and a clinical sensitivity of 95%. When compared with the previously available NucliSENS ASR, both assays showed excellent sensitivity.[40] The MultiCode-PLx RUO assay has reported sensitivity of 100%; however only a small number of positive samples were tested.[21,23] The ResPlex II Panel RUO assay has a significantly lower sensitivity of 80%.[22] There are few reports of in-house developed assays for metapneumovirus, and those suffer from low number of positive samples and lack of a comparator assay.[14,41]

OTHER RESPIRATORY VIRUSES

Viruses previously considered to be upper respiratory pathogens such as rhinoviruses and coronaviruses (CoVs) more recently have been reported to play a role in respiratory hospitalizations also. Rhinoviruses classically have been associated with URIs, including the common cold, otitis media, and sinusitis, causing illnesses throughout the year but with peaks in early fall and spring.[42] The clinical significance and precise role of rhinoviruses in LRI in healthy hosts need further investigation. No assay is approved by the FDA for detecting rhinovirus. All three assays employing multiplex PCR and fluid microsphere-based array detection on the Luminex x-MAP system include rhinovirus as a target. The xTAG Respiratory Virus Panel has an analytical sensitivity of 3×10^{-2} $TCID_{50}$/mL and clinical sensitivity and specificity of 100% and 91%, respectively.[33] The MultiCode-PLx also had a sensitivity of 100%, with some false-positive results.[35] In-house developed assays employing NASBA and RT-PCR showed sensitivities of 85% and 83%, respectively. Both assays were significantly more sensitive than culture (45%).[43] There appear to be rhinoviruses that are not detected using these molecular methods and positive results that cannot be confirmed by culture. More sequence data from different rhinovirus serotypes and currently circulating strains are needed to improve primer coverage.

Five CoV species have been described to cause human disease. CoV-229E and CoV-OC43, described in the 1960s are causative agents of the common cold and LRIs in young children and elderly adults.[44,45] Severe acute respiratory syndrome CoV (SARS-CoV), the causative agent of an outbreak of SARS worldwide from 2002 to 2003 has not been found to circulate in people since 2004. Two new CoVs, however, CoV-NL63 and CoV-HKU1, were described in 2004 and 2005 respectively. These viruses, although newly discovered, subsequently have been shown to have been circulating in people for a long time. These new CoVs have been associated with both URIs and LRIs.[46] No assay is approved by the FDA for detecting CoV. The xTAG Respiratory Virus Panel is not FDA-approved for CoV but has been used to study the epidemiology of the virus. It has an analytical sensitivity of 50 genome equivalents.[33] The MultiCode-PLx RUO assay includes CoVs except for HKU1. Published reports suffer from inadequate number of positive specimens to assess performance.[34]

Bocavirus, a new virus discovered in 2005 using nonspecific nucleic acid amplification techniques, has been detected in 2% to 19% of samples from patients with acute respiratory symptoms.[47] Limited sequence data are available for bocavirus, making selection of conserved regions difficult. Detection using real-time PCR methods, however, has been used to detect bocavirus.[48] Although an increasing number of studies have reported detection of bocavirus in patients who have respiratory illnesses, determination of a causal relationship in LRI has been difficult given:

The high rates of codetection of other respiratory pathogens
Prolonged detection in some patients raising questions about possible persistence or prolonged infections
Lack of cell culture or serodiagnostic methods that could help differentiate true infection from nucleic acid detection

CONSIDERATIONS FOR IN-HOUSE DEVELOPED ASSAYS
Extraction

An important, yet underemphasized aspect of nucleic acid amplification-based diagnostic methods is the extraction system used. Detection of respiratory viruses cannot be performed adequately without specimen extraction.[49,50] Respiratory viruses are predominantly RNA genomes; however, adenovirus and bocavirus are DNA viruses that should be included in a diagnostic screening assay. An extract that contains total nucleic acids is most useful for that type of application. Different systems have differing abilities to recover RNA, DNA, or total nucleic acids.[40,51–54] When determining the performance characteristics of laboratory-developed assays or assays employing ASRs, the performance characteristics of the extraction system also must be documented. FDA-approved kits are approved using a specific method of extraction. Use of a different method by a laboratory requires the user to perform a complete revalidation of the performance characteristics of the kit.

Primer and Probe Design

There are numerous reports in the literature of laboratory-developed assays for detecting respiratory viruses. Many of these reports include the target gene; some include the amino acid position, and few include in silico coverage rates for the primers and probes described.[55] The amplification and detection format employed will determine the number of mismatches permissible while still retaining target detection. It is mportant to check the coverage regularly to ensure that newly emerging strains can be detected.

Amplification Method

PCR or RT-PCR are the most commonly used nucleic acid amplification methods for detecting respiratory viruses; many of these employ primers to a single target. Design of multiplex assays requires good primer design and extensive validation to document lack of interference. There are reports of in-house developed multiplex assays and commercially available products. The implementation of touchdown amplification protocols that involve a stepped reduction in the annealing temperature, which introduces an advantage for specific binding, allows for multiplexing and a common amplification protocol.[56] Isothermal amplification procedures such as NASBA[16,40] and LAMP[57] also have been used for detecting respiratory viruses.

Detection

Real-time detection eliminates the manipulation of amplified products, which minimizes problems associated with amplicon, contamination, carryover, and false-positive reactions. It also decreases the turnaround time of the assays. Real-time detection most often employs target specific probes, thus also increasing the specificity of the assay. Various probe chemistries and labels are available. The choice of probe format and label often is determined by the detection platform employed. Spectral overlap of fluorescent labels, however, also limits the number of multiplex target detection options. Thus, real-time detection is extremely useful; however, it is not adaptable to broad range multianalyte screening.

To improve amplification efficiency and expand multiplexing ability, postamplification detection must be employed. Postamplification detection requires handling of amplicon and significantly increasing turn around time. The advantage is the ability to detect multiple pathogens in a single assay. Because of the large number of viruses capable of causing similar symptoms in patients, the diagnosis of respiratory tract infections seems uniquely suited for this application. Solid-phase microarrays allow for a large number of probes to be employed and also may allow for variable hybridization conditions such that detection of a large number of targets or mismatched targets can be accomplished. Suspension microarrays employ a liquid phase bead conjugated array. These allow for rapid hybridization conditions and flexibility in assay design. Bead makeup can be modified easily. Although no automated microarray system is approved by the FDA, these systems have the potential to decrease hands on technologist time; however, it currently is at the cost of turnaround time.[21]

REFERENCES

1. Henrickson KJ, Hoover S, Kehl SC, et al. National disease burden of respiratory viruses detected in children by polymerase chain reaction. Pediatr Infect Dis J 2004;24(Suppl 1):S11–8.
2. Barenfanger J, Drake C, Leon N, et al. Clinical and financial benefits of rapid detection of respiratory viruses: an outcomes study. J Clin Microbiol 2000; 38(8):2824–8.
3. Woo PCY, Chiu SS, Seto W, et al. Cost-effectiveness of rapid diagnosis of viral respiratory tract infections in pediatric patients. J Clin Microbiol 1997;35(6): 1579–81.

4. US Department of Health and Human Services. Guidance for industry and FDA staff. Commercially distributed analyte-specific reagents (ASRs): frequently asked questions. Document No.1590. Federal Register 2007;72(178):52568–70.
5. Poehling KA, Edwards KM, Weinberg GA, et al. New Vaccine Surveillance Network. The under-recognized burden of influenza in young children. N Engl J Med 2006;355(1):31–40.
6. Thompson WW, Shay DK, Weintraub E, et al. Influenza-associated hospitalizations in the United States. J Am Med Assoc 2004;292(11):1333–40.
7. Steininger C, Kundi M, Aberle SW, et al. Effectiveness of reverse transcription PCR, virus isolation, and enzyme-linked immunosorbent assay for diagnosis of influenza A virus infection in different age groups. J Clin Microbiol 2002;40(6): 2051–6.
8. Hindiyeh M, Hillyard DR, Carroll KC. Evaluation of the Prodesse Hexaplex multiplex PCR assay for direct detection of seven respiratory viruses in clinical specimens. Am J Clin Pathol 2001;116:218–24.
9. Fan J, Henrickson KJ, Savatski LL. Rapid simultaneous diagnosis of infections with respiratory syncytial viruses A and B, influenza A and B, and human parainfluenza virus types 1, 2, and 3 by multiplex quantitative reverse transcription-polymerase chain reaction-enzyme hybridization (Hexaplex) assay. Clin Infect Dis 1998;26:1397–402.
10. Mahony J, Chong S, Merante F, et al. Development of a respiratory virus panel test for detection of twenty human respiratory viruses by use of multiplex PCR and a fluid microbead-based assay. J Clin Microbiol 2007;45(9):2965–70.
11. Krunic N, Yager TD, Himsworth D, et al. xTAG TM RSV assay: analytical and clinical performance. J Clin Virol 2007;40(Suppl 1):S39–46.
12. Kehl SC, Henrickson KJ, Hua W, et al. Evaluation of the Hexaplex assay for detection of respiratory viruses in children. J Clin Microbiol 2001;39(5):1696–701.
13. Ruest A, Michaud S, Deslandes S, et al. Comparison of the Directogen flu A+B test, the QuickVue influenza test, and clinical case definition to viral culture and reverse transcription PCR for rapid diagnosis of influenza virus infection. J Clin Microbiol 2003;41(8):3487–93.
14. Kuypers J, Wright N, Ferrenberg J, et al. Comparison of real-time PCR assays with fluorescent antibody assays for diagnosis of respiratory virus infections in children. J Clin Microbiol 2006;44(7):2382–8.
15. Habib-Bein NF, Beckwith WH, Mayo D, et al. Comparison of Smartcycler real-time reverse transcription PCR assay in a public health laboratory with direct immunofluorescence and cell culture assays in a medical center for detection of influenza A virus. J Clin Microbiol 2003;41(8):3597–601.
16. Moore C, Hibbitts S, Owen N, et al. Development and evaluation of a real-time nucleic acid sequence-based amplification assay for rapid detection of influenza A. J Med Virol 2004;74:619–28.
17. LeGoff J, Kara R, Moulin F, et al. Evaluation of the one-step multiplex real-time reverse transcription PCR ProFlu—an assay for detection of influenza A and influenza B viruses and respiratory syncytial viruses in children. J Clin Microbiol 2008; 46(2):789–91.
18. van Elden LJ, van Kraaij MG, Nijhuis M, et al. Polymerase chain reactions is more sensitive than viral culture and antigen testing for the detection of respiratory viruses in adults with hematological cancer and pneumonia. Clinical Infectious Diseases 2002;34:177–83.
19. van Kraaij MG, van Elden LJ, van Loon AM, et al. Frequent detection of respiratory viruses in adult recipients of stem cell transplants with the use of real-time

polymerase chain reaction, compared with viral culture. Clin Infect Dis 2005; 40(5):662–9.

20. Weinberg A, Zamora MR, Li S, et al. The value of polymerase chain reaction for the diagnosis of viral respiratory tract infections in lung transplant recipients. J Clin Virol 2002;25(2):171–5.
21. Marshall DJ, Reisdorf E, Harms G, et al. Evaluation of a multiplexed PCR assay for detection of respiratory viral pathogens in a public health laboratory setting. J Clin Microbiol 2007;45(12):3875–82.
22. Li H, McCormac MA, Estes RW, et al. Simultaneous detection and high-throughput identification of a panel of RNA viruses causing respiratory tract infections. J Clin Microbiol 2007;45(7):2105–9.
23. Nolte FS, Marshall DJ, Rasberry C, et al. MultiCode-PLx system for multiplexed detection of seventeen respiratory viruses. J Clin Microbiol 2007;45(9):2779–86.
24. Raymond F, Carbonneau J, Boucher N, et al. Comparison of automated microarray detection with real-time PCR assays for detection of respiratory viruses in specimens obtained from children. J Clin Microbiol 2009;47(3):743–50.
25. Hall CB, Weinberg A, Iwane MK, et al. The burden of respiratory syncytial virus infection in young children. N Engl J Med 2009;360(6):588–98.
26. Falsey AR, Hennessey PA, Formica MA, et al. Respiratory syncytial virus infection in elderly and high-risk adults. N Engl J Med 2005;352:1749–59.
27. Liao RS, Tomalty LL, Majury A, et al. Comparison of viral isolation and multiplex real-time reverse transcription PCR for confirmation of respiratory syncytial virus and influenza virus detection by antigen immunoassays. J Clin Microbiol 2009; 47(3):527–32.
28. Goodrich JS, Miller MB. Comparison of Cepheid's analyte-specific reagents with BD Directigen for detection of respiratory syncytial virus. J Clin Microbiol 2007; 45(2):604–6.
29. Boivin G, Cote S, Dery P, et al. Multiplex real-time PCR assay for detection of influenza and human respiratory syncytial viruses. J Clin Microbiol 2004;42(1):45–51.
30. Hu A, Colella M, Tam JS, et al. Simultaneous detection, subgrouping, and quantitation of respiratory syncytial virus A and B by real-time PCR. J Clin Microbiol 2003;41(1):149–54.
31. Erdman DD, Weinberg GA, Edwards KM, et al. GeneScan reverse transcription PCR assay for detection of six common respiratory viruses in young children hospitalized with acute respiratory illness. J Clin Microbiol 2003;41(9):4298–303.
32. van Elden LJ, van Loon AM, van der Beek A, et al. Applicability of a real-time quantitative PCR assay for diagnosis of respiratory syncytial virus infection in immunocompromised adults. J Clin Microbiol 2003;41(9):4378–81.
33. Mahony JB. Detection of respiratory viruses by molecular methods. Clin Microbiol Rev 2008;21(4):716–47.
34. Lee WM, Grindle K, Pappas T, et al. High-throughput, sensitive, and accurate multiplex PCR-microsphere flow cytometry system for large-scale comprehensive detection of respiratory viruses. J Clin Microbiol 2007;45(8):2626–34.
35. Henrickson KJ. Parainfluenza viruses. Clinical Microbiology Reviews 2003;16(2): 242–64.
36. Templeton KE, Scheltinga SA, Beersma MFC, et al. Rapid and sensitive method using multiplex real-time PCR for diagnosis of infections by influenza A and influenza B viruses, respiratory syncytial virus, and parainfluenza viruses 1, 2, 3, and 4. J Clin Microbiol 2004;42(4):1564–9.
37. Echavarria M. Adenoviruses in immunocompromised hosts. Clinical Microbiology Reviews 2008;21:704–15.

38. Williams JV, Harris PA, Tollefson SJ, et al. Human metapneumovirus and lower respiratory tract disease in otherwise healthy infants and children. N Engl J Med 2004;350:443–50.
39. Williams JV. Human metapneumovirus: an important cause of respiratory disease in children and adults. Current Infectious Disease Report 2005;7(3):204–10.
40. Ginocchio CC, Manji R, Lotlikar M, et al. Clinical evaluation of NucliSENS magnetic extraction and NucliSENS analyte-specific reagents for real-time detection of human metapneumovirus in pediatric respiratory specimens. J Clin Microbiol 2008;46(4):1274–80.
41. Gruteke P, Glas AS, Dierdorp M, et al. Practical implementation of a multiplex PCR for acute respiratory tract infections in children. J Clin Microbiol 2004; 42(12):5596–603.
42. Hayden FG. Rhinovirus and the lower respiratory tract. Rev Med Virol 2004;14: 17–31.
43. Loens K, Goossens H, de Laat C, et al. Detection of rhinoviruses by tissue culture and two independent amplification techniques, nucleic acid sequence-based amplification and reverse transcription PCR, in children with acute respiratory infections during a winter season. J Clin Microbiol 2006;44(1):166–71.
44. Falsey AR, Walsh EE, Hayden FG. Rhinovirus and coronavirus infection-associated hospitalization among older adults. J Infect Dis 2002;185(9):1338–41.
45. van der Hoek L, Pyrc K, Berkhout B. Human coronavirus NL63, a new respiratory virus. FEMS Microbiol Rev 2006;30(5):760–73.
46. Kuypers J, Martin ET, Heugel J, et al. Clinical disease in children associated with newly described coronavirus subtypes. Pediatrics 2007;119(1):e70–6.
47. Schildgen O, Muller A, Allander T, et al. Human bocavirus: passenger or pathogen in acute respiratory tract infections? Clin Microbiol Rev 2008;21(2): 291–304.
48. Lu X, Chittaganpitch M, Olsen SJ, et al. Real-time PCR assays for detection of bocavirus in human specimens. J Clin Microbiol 2006;44(9):3231–5.
49. Claas EC, van Milaan AJ, Sprenger MJW, et al. Prospective application of reverse transcriptase polymerase chain reaction for diagnosing influenza infections in respiratory samples from a children's hospital. J Clin Microbiol 1993;31(8): 2218–21.
50. Letant SE, Ortiz JI, Bentley Tammero LF, et al. Multiplexed reverse transcriptase PCR assay for identification of viral respiratory pathogens at the point of care. J Clin Microbiol 2007;45(11):3498–505.
51. Chan KH, Yam WC, Pan CM, et al. Comparison of the NucliSens easyMAG and Qiagne BioRobot 9604 nucleic acid extraction systems for detection of RNA and DNA respiratory viruses in nasopharyngeal aspirate samples. J Clin Microbiol 2008;46(7):2195–9.
52. Kehl SC, Vuaghn K. Evaluation of the NucliSens EasyMag for the extraction of influenza A/V, respiratory syncytial virus, and herpes simplex virus for use in Smartcycler assays. Presented at the 22nd Annual Clinical Virology Symposium. Clearwater Beach (FL): 2006.
53. Kehl SC, Goodacre S, Vaughn K, et al. Comparison of the Jaguar system, the Qiagen Biorobot EZ1, and the Nuclisens easyMAG for extraction of enterovirus, RSV, influenza A, and HSV 1 and 2. Presented at the 25th Annual Clinical Virology Symposium. Daytona Beach (FL): 2009.
54. Loens K, Bergs K, Ursi D, et al. Evaluation of NucliSens easyMAG for automated nucleic acid extraction from various clinical specimens. J Clin Microbiol 2007; 45(2):421–5.

55. Bose M, Beck ET, Ledeboer N, et al. Rapid semiautomated subtyping of influenza during the 2009 swine-origin influenza A H1N1 virus epidemic in Milwaukee, Wisconsin. Published ahead of print 2009 July 29. J Clin Microbiol 2009. doi:10.1128/JCM.00999.09.

56. Coyle PV, Ong GM, O'Neill HJ, et al. A touchdown nucleic acid amplification protocol as an alternative to culture backup for immunofluorescence in the routine diagnosis of acute viral respiratory tract infections. BMC Microbiol 2004;4:41–9.

57. Poon LLM, Leung CSW, Chan KH, et al. Detection of human influenza A viruses by loop-mediated isothermal amplification. J Clin Microbiol 2005;43(1):427–30.

Emerging Molecular Assays for Detection and Characterization of Respiratory Viruses

Wenjuan Wu, PhD[a,c], Yi-Wei Tang, MD, PhD[a,b,d],*

KEYWORDS

- Respiratory viruses • Quantum dots
- In vitro nucleic acid amplification • Multiplex • Pyrosequencing
- Padlock probes • Microarrays • Mass spectrometry

Rapid detection and identification of viral pathogens causing respiratory tract infections is critical for initiating antiviral therapy, avoiding unnecessary antimicrobial therapy, preventing nosocomial spread, decreasing the duration of hospitalization, and reducing management costs. Molecular assays, which provide high sensitivity and specificity, short test turnaround time, and automatic, high-throughput batch processing, have played critical roles in rapid detection, screening, and identification of emerging respiratory viral pathogens, such as severe acute respiratory syndrome coronavirus (SARS-CoV) and novel A/H1N1 influenza (Flu) virus.[1–3] The superiority of polymerase chain reaction (PCR), reverse transcription-PCR (RT-PCR), and other in vitro nucleic acid amplification assays over conventional methods for the diagnosis of respiratory viral infections has already been established.[4,5] This article describes several emerging molecular assays that have potential applications in the diagnosis and monitoring of respiratory viral infections.

DIRECT NUCLEIC ACID DETECTION BY QUANTUM DOTS BIOSENSORS

Biosensors offer the possibility of real-time monitoring, and the deployment of these devices in the field would provide a means for prompt etiologic diagnosis. All

[a] Department of Pathology, Vanderbilt University Medical Center, 4605 TVC, 1161 21st South Avenue, Nashville, TN, USA
[b] Department of Medicine, Vanderbilt University Medical Center, 4605 TVC, 1161 21st South Avenue, Nashville, TN, USA
[c] Shanghai Public Health Clinical Center, Fudan University, 2901 Caolang Road, Shanghai, 201508, People's Republic of China
[d] Molecular Infectious Disease Laboratory, Vanderbilt University Hospital, 4605 TVC, Nashville, TN 37232-5310, USA
* Corresponding author. Molecular Infectious Disease Laboratory, Vanderbilt University Hospital, 4605 TVC, Nashville, TN 37232-5310.
E-mail address: yiwei.tang@vanderbilt.edu (Y.W. Tang).

Clin Lab Med 29 (2009) 673–693
doi:10.1016/j.cll.2009.07.005
0272-2712/09/$ – see front matter © 2009 Elsevier Inc. All rights reserved.

labmed.theclinics.com

biosensors are essentially composed of a biologic recognition element or bioreceptor, which interacts with the analyte and responds in some manner that can be registered by a transducer. The bioreceptor is a crucial component, and its function is to impart selectivity so that the sensor responds only to a particular analyte or biomolecule of interest, hence avoiding interference from other substances. The transducer converts the microbial biorecognition event into an electrical signal detected using electro-chemical, optical, or piezoelectric platforms.[6,7] A biosensor specifically targeting nucleic acids through hybridization is called a genosensor. Genosensors have been used to for direct, on-demand, and real-time detection and discrimination of microbial pathogens in clinical specimens. Malamud and colleagues[8] developed a group of genosensor-based assays to detect microbial pathogens in oral specimens for use in the diagnosis of multiple infectious diseases. A piezoelectric DNA biosensor to directly detect hepatitis B virus was developed based on the mass-transducing function of a quartz crystal microbalance and nucleic acid hybridization[9]; another hybridization-based amperometric biosensor, using osmium as an electrochemical indicator, was used for the detection and confirmation of virus-specific PCR products.[10] A generic semidisposable fluorescence biosensor was developed to directly detect dengue virus RNA.[11] A hybridization-based genosensor on gold film coupled with enzymatic electrochemical detection was designed to detect SARS-CoV RNA.[12]

Fluorescent semiconductor nanocrystals, known as quantum dots (Qdots), are colloidal particles consisting of a semiconductor core, a high band gap material shell, and typically an outer coating layer. The core-size–dependent photoluminescence with narrow emission bandwidths that span the visible spectrum and the broad adsorption spectra allow simultaneous excitation of mixed Qdot populations at a single wavelength. Qdots also exhibit several unique features: high quantum yield, high resistance to photodegradation, and better near-infrared emission.[13,14] The new generation of Qdots has far-reaching potential for the study of intracellular processes in broad fields, including diagnostics.[14] High-sensitivity bacterial detection using biotin-tagged phage and quantum-dot nanocomplexes has been described, which provides specific limits of detection at 10 bacterial cells/mL in 1 hour.[15] A bead-based microfluidic device was developed to achieve an ELISA with Qdots as the labeling fluorophore for virus detection.[16] Three groups have reported the use of Qdots conjugated to specific monoclonal antibodies to detect and identify the presence of respiratory syncytial virus (RSV) in a real-time manner, implying that Qdots may provide a method for early, rapid detection of RSV infections.[17–19] In addition to microbial pathogen antigen detection, positively charged compact Qdot-DNA complexes were described that can detect H5N1 Flu-A virus nucleic acids presented at concentrations as low as 200 nmol.[20] Simultaneous excitation of several emission-tunable Qdot populations can be combined with a pool of differentially labeled probes for multiplex target analysis.[21,22] Qdot-based techniques are under development to detect a panel of respiratory viruses, producing more efficient assays that require smaller quantities of target nucleic acids.

AMPLIFICATION METHODS AND PLATFORMS
Loop-Mediated Isothermal Amplification

First described by Notomi and colleagues[23] in 2000, loop-mediated isothermal amplification (LAMP) is a simple, rapid, and specific nucleic acid amplification method, which is characterized by the use of multiple primers specifically designed to recognize several distinct regions on the target gene. Amplification and detection of target genes can be completed in a single step, by incubating the mixture of samples, primers, DNA polymerase with strand displacement activity and substrates at a constant temperature. Because amplification is isothermal, LAMP does not require special reagents or sophisticated temperature control devices. Because the increase in turbidity of the reaction mixture according to the production of precipitate correlates with the amount of DNA synthesized, real-time monitoring of the LAMP reaction can be achieved by turbidity measurement.[24] With a detection limit of about one to two copies, LAMP is capable of detecting the presence of pathogenic agents earlier than PCR if the gene copy number is low.[25]

LAMP has successfully been applied to the rapid and real-time detection of several emerging and reemerging human pathogens, including West Nile virus, dengue virus, Japanese encephalitis virus, monkey pox virus, Rift Valley virus, SARS-CoV, Chikungunya virus, and noroviruses.[25-28] Poon and colleagues[29] described the use of an RT-LAMP to detect Flu-A viruses covering H1 to H3. Another similar RT-LAMP assay was described more recently that detects Flu-A virus H1 and H3 subtype strains and Flu-B virus strains.[30] At a limit of detection of 10 focus-forming units per mL, both assays can be completed within 3 hours, providing rapid and sensitive detection.[29,30] Two one-step RT-LAMP assays with analytical sensitivities of 0.01 to 0.1 plaque-forming units (pfu) per reaction were developed specifically for detection of highly pathogenic avian Flu-A (H5N1) viruses and validated using H5N1 viral strains isolated over the past 10 years and clinical specimens.[31-33] An RT-LAMP assay was reported to specifically detect the H9 subtype of avian Flu virus with a detection limit of 10 copies per reaction, 10-fold lower than that of RT-PCR.[34] In Japan, the LAMP assay was used to rapidly subtype Flu-A virus and confirm two cases of influenza in patients who had returned from Thailand.[30]

In addition to the detection and typing of Flu viruses, a subgroup-A/B–specific RT-LAMP assay was developed to amplify RSV to improve current diagnostic methods for RSV infections. The assay was validated using nasopharyngeal aspirates from children who had respiratory tract infections, and the results indicated that the RT-LAMP is more sensitive than viral isolation and antigen testing for RSV detection.[35,36] Several LAMP-based assays were reported for rapid detection of SARS-CoV with the advantages of rapid amplification, simple operation, and ease of detection.[28,37] LAMP-based assays have also been used to detect other respiratory viral pathogens, such as mumps,[38,39] measles,[40] and adenoviruses.[41] In comparison to conventional RT-PCR, RT-LAMP assays demonstrated 10- to 100-fold enhanced sensitivity, with a detection limit of 0.01 to 10 pfu of virus in most cases.

Multiplex Ligation-Dependent Probe Amplification

Recently established in The Netherlands, multiplex ligation-dependent probe amplification (MLPA) makes use of both ligation and PCR.[42] Inventively modified from previously described ligation-dependent PCR assays,[43,44] the MLPA platform features greatly reduced probe concentrations and longer hybridization periods to generate conditions compatible with multiplex analysis. Each MLPA probe consists of a pair of oligonucleotides subject to ligation when hybridized to a target sequence, analogous to a padlock probe (see later discussion). One oligonucleotide consists of a 5′ fluorescent label, a universal forward primer binding site, and a target-specific recognition sequence at the 3′ end, whereas the other oligonucleotide consists of a target-specific recognition sequence at the 5′ end, a nonspecific stretch of DNA of defined length ("stuffer" sequence), and a universal reverse primer binding site at the 3′ end. Each MLPA assay is divided into three basic steps: (1) annealing of probes to their target sequences, (2) ligation of the probes, and (3) PCR amplification of ligated probes using universal primers. Multiplexing is achieved by varying the length of stuffer sequence for each unique set of probes used in the assay. Amplification products are detected using high-resolution electrophoretic techniques, such as capillary electrophoresis, and it is claimed that this approach allows relative quantification.[42]

MLPA-based techniques have proved sufficiently sensitive, reproducible, and sequence specific for use in screening human DNA. Recent studies have use of the MLPA assay for the detection and identification of several pathogenic microorganisms, including rapid characterization of *Mycobacterium tuberculosis*,[45] and relative quantification of targeted bacterial species in oral microbiota.[46] Reijans and colleagues[47] described an MLPA technology–based RespiFinder assay to detect 15 respiratory viruses simultaneously in one reaction. In this case, the MLPA reaction was preceded by a preamplification step that ensured detection of both RNA and DNA viruses with the same specificity and sensitivity as individual monoplex real-time RT-PCR assays. The RespiFinder assay showed satisfactory specificity and perfect sensitivity for adenovirus, human metapneumovirus (hMPV), Flu-A, parainfluenza virus (PIV) types 1 and 3, rhinovirus (RhV), and RSV. Use of the RespiFinder assay resulted in a 24.5% increase in the diagnostic yield compared with cell culture. This assay is being extended to cover four additional bacterial pathogens that cause respiratory tract infections: *Mycoplasma pneumoniae*, *Chlamydophila pneumoniae*, *Legionella pneumophila*, and *Bordetella pertussis*.

Polymerase Chain Reaction Amplification Using Arbitrary Primers

PCR amplification techniques using arbitrary primers, including arbitrarily primed (AP) PCR,[48] sequence-independent single-primer amplification (SISPA),[49] and randomly amplified polymorphic DNA (RAPD),[50] are generally based on the PCR amplification of random DNA segments with short primers (usually a single 1 of 10 nucleotides) containing arbitrary nucleotide sequences. RAPD-based assays have increasingly been used to type microorganisms, especially during clinical outbreaks.[51] The RAPD-PCR technique seems to be practical and efficient for routine use in high-resolution viral diversity studies by providing assemblage comparisons through fingerprinting, probing, or sequence information.[52] Similar techniques have been used to characterize the polymerase gene and genomic termini of Nipah virus[53] and avian Flu virus genome sequences.[54]

On the other hand, AP-PCR and SISPA-based assays have mainly been used for the discovery and characterization of novel and noncultivatable viruses.[55] Because viral pathogens do not possess conserved, universal genes, such as 16S rRNA genes, SISPA was used in the early 1990s as a random PCR amplification strategy to amplify known and unknown viral genes, including those of hepatitis C virus, rotavirus, and norovirus.[56–58] The AP-PCR technique was used successfully to obtain sequence information on a novel hMPV after the virus was cultured.[59] Wang and colleagues[60,61] used a similar random amplification technique in conjunction with a long oligonucleotide pan-viral microarray to simultaneously screen and detect hundreds of viral pathogens. This system has successfully been used for the detection of a human PIV-4 strain associated with respiratory failure,[62] for identification of a novel gammaretrovirus in a patient who had prostate tumors,[63] for the diagnosis of a critical respiratory illness caused by hMPV,[64] and for the identification of cardioviruses related to Theiler murine encephalomyelitis virus in human infections.[65] Quan and colleagues[66] recently reported the use of a similar random amplification process followed by comprehensive microarray analysis (GreeneChipResp) to detect diverse respiratory viral pathogens and subtype Flu-A viruses.

A modified SISPA incorporating DNAse treatment has recently been used to discover, identify, and characterize several novel bovine and human viral pathogens directly from clinical samples.[67–70] The same technology has been used for the characterization of common epitopes in enterovirus (EnV),[71] identification of a novel human coronavirus,[72] detection of TT virus in stool samples collected during a gastroenteritis outbreak,[73] and discovery of novel unculturable viruses in specimens collected from patients presenting with fever of unknown origin.[74,75] Although PCR amplification using arbitrary primers has been an extremely powerful approach for screening and discovery of new or noncultivable viral pathogens directly from clinical specimens, subsequent identification and confirmation steps are hindered by a background of nonspecific random amplification products. Further development is thus required to optimize this technology for routine diagnostic use in molecular microbiology laboratories.

Target-Enriched Multiplexing Amplification

Multiplex PCR was developed to use numerous primers within a single reaction tube to amplify nucleic acid fragments from different targets. Multiple sets of high-concentration primers in the conventional multiplex reaction often favor primer-dimer formation, however, resulting in nonspecific amplification. To meet the challenges of conventional multiplex PCR, Han and colleagues[76] developed target-enriched multiplexing (TEM)-PCR technology, which uses nested gene-specific primers at extremely low concentrations to enrich specific targets during early PCR cycles and relies on universal forward and reverse "superprimers" at high, but unequal, concentrations to achieve exponential asymmetric target amplification. TEM-PCR amplification has been reported for the detection, typing, and semiquantification of 25 human papillomaviruses,[76] detection and differentiation of a panel of respiratory bacterial pathogens,[77–79] detection and differentiation of 24 antituberculosis drug resistance-related mutations,[80] determination of antibiotic resistance and detection of toxin-encoding genes in *Staphylococcus aureus*,[81] screening and differentiation of methicillin-resistant *S aureus* and vancomycin-resistant enterococci,[82] and characterization and typing of Flu-A, including H5N1.[83]

Using TEM technology, the ResPlex II assay was developed to detect Flu-A, Flu-B, PIV-1, PIV-2, PIV-3, PIV-4, RSV, hMPV, RhV, EnV, and SARS-CoV in a single reaction.[78,84,85] When monoplex RT PCR is used for pathogen detection, the clinician often does not consider the possible presence of other pathogens when given a positive result. The multiplex approach offered by the ResPlex II system enhances diagnosis through detection of respiratory viral etiologic agents in cases in which their presence was unsuspected and an appropriate test consequently was not ordered by the clinician.[85] A recent study by Brunstein and colleagues[84] revealed that, using the ResPlex II kit covering 12 viral pathogens, 2.5% of specimens were coinfected with two or three different viruses. (A low level of cross-reactivity between PIV-1 and PIV-3 was noticed using this assay.[85]) These coinfections are medically relevant, and effective treatment of severe respiratory tract infections will increasingly require diagnosis of all involved pathogens, as opposed to single-pathogen reporting.[84] The original ResPlex II system detects only RNA viruses, but adenoviruses, bocavirus, and four coronaviruses have been added to a recently released new version of ResPlex II. Preliminary data indicate that the overall sensitivity and specificity of ResPlex II v2.0 is comparable to that of the ResPlex II panel. A notable number of previously negative samples were found to be positive for one of the newly added bocavirus or coronavirus targets (John Brunstein, 2009; personal communication). A factor that could diminish the analytical and clinical performance of ResPlex II and ResPlex II v2.0 is the potential for false-positive results caused by carryover of PCR products using the Luminex platform.

AMPLIFICATION PRODUCT DETECTION AND IDENTIFICATION
Pyrosequencing

Direct amplicon sequencing provides simple, rapid, and accurate means of detection and identification of amplification products. The need for robust, high-throughput methods to replace the elegant Sanger method, which was described more than 30 years ago,[86] has led to the development of several new principles. Ronaghi and colleagues[87,88] described in 1998 a pyrosequencing technique, a non–gel-based real-time approach to sequencing DNA by monitoring DNA polymerase activity. Pyrosequencing is based on enzymatic inorganic pyrophosphate release by DNA polymerase. This reaction is stoichiometric; the amount of light produced is proportional to the number of pyrophosphate molecules generated and, hence, the number of incorporated nucleotides. Unincorporated nucleotides are degraded with apyrase before the next nucleotide is added. In this way, sequence information on an interrogated region is generated quantitatively in real time. Although basic approaches to performing pyrosequencing remain the same, numerous commercial systems have been used widely to rapidly identify infectious agents and screen for antimicrobial drug resistance.[89–91] Multiplexed pyrosequencing involving the simultaneous extension of several primers hybridized to one or more target DNA templates[92] has gained broad acceptance in the fields of cytogenetics, pharmacogenetics, and medical genetics.[71,93,94]

Most applications of pyrosequencing in the identification and characterization of respiratory viruses have focused on Flu-A. Based on pyrosequencing technology, a rapid and highly informative diagnostic assay was reported for the detection of H5N1 Flu viruses[95]; sequencing of critical regions within the H5 virus was developed as a screening method during high volumes of H5N1 activity.[95] A real-time RT-PCR pyrosequencing assay was developed that combines restriction enzyme digestion and direct sequencing to screen and verify H5 Flu infections in humans.[96] Another RT-PCR assay with subsequent pyrosequencing analysis allows for a rapid, high-throughput, and cost-effective screening of subtype A/H1N1, A/H3N2, and A/H5N1 viruses and can clearly discriminate wild-type from a mutant viruses.[97] A study reported by Bright and colleagues[98] showed an alarming increase in the incidence of amantadine- and rimantadine-resistant H3N2 Flu-A viruses worldwide when the pyrosequencing technique was configured to cover a 44–base pair region of the M2 protein-encoding gene. Pyrosequencing assay capabilities were expanded to screen for 52 amino acid changes defined as avian or human specific,[99] and pyrosequencing-based assays recently were designed for detection and surveillance of the most commonly reported mutations associated with resistance to neuraminidase inhibitors and the adamantanes.[100–106] The latter detects mutations associated with resistance directly in clinical specimens, thus reducing the time required for testing and avoiding selection of novel sequence variants by cell culture. In addition, pyrosequencing-based assays have been reported for the characterization, quantification, typing, subtyping, and drug-resistance profiling of other viruses.[107–112]

One unique feature of pyrosequencing is its theoretical adaptability to the analysis of any genetic marker, which allows for the detection of multiple known and unknown mutations in a single pyrosequencing reaction. Integration of high-throughput pyrosequencing with the Roche/454 instrument has become a powerful tool for whole genome sequencing without the need for additional equipment or molecular techniques other than standard PCR, Genome Sequencer FLX sample preparation, and the sequencing pipeline.[113] Pyrosequencing generates sequence content quantitatively, which has made pyrosequencing a primary choice for quantifying specific mutations (eg, detection of drug resistance–associated signatures) in mixed genomic populations. Because pyrosequencing byproducts inhibit the sequencing reaction, pyrosequencing read lengths are limited to less than 100 base pairs. Another drawback of pyrosequencing-based techniques includes secondary structure formation, which affects quality of the results, particularly with GC-rich targets. Additionally, it may be difficult to determine the precise number of nucleotides in a homopolymeric region based on peak heights.[87] It is expected that pyrosequencing-based diagnostic devices will soon become available for rapid characterization and typing of viral pathogens.

Padlock Probes

Padlock probes, originated by Nilsson and colleagues[114] in 1994, are linear oligonucleotides designed so that the two end segments, connected by a linker region, are both complementary to a target sequence. On hybridization to a target sequence, the two probe ends become juxtaposed and can be joined by a DNA ligase. Reacted probes can be detected by way of reporter molecules attached to the linker.[115] Alternatively, an amplified signal can be obtained from the circularized probes by rolling circle amplification. Padlock probes provide a means for detection and quantification of large numbers of DNA or RNA sequences and for highly multiplexed genetic studies.[116] The application of padlock probes for the detection of microbial pathogens is a recent trend in molecular diagnoses.[117]

The unique padlock probe design provides the benefit of speed and sensitivity derived from using a nucleic acid–based method, and the amount of information is greatly increased by extensive multiplexing. Indeed, this method was used to simultaneously detect and type 16 HA and 9 NA subtypes of avian Flu virus. The analysis is completed within approximately 4 hours and performed in a single reaction tube, which helps to decrease the risk for contamination, with just a few sequential additions of reagents before the readout is performed using an oligonucleotide array.[118] Padlock probes combined with back-end microarray technology have been developed to detect foot-and-mouth disease, vesicular stomatitis, and swine vesicular disease viruses.[119] Besides viral pathogens, padlock probe–based techniques have been rapidly extended in recent years to the identification and characterization of bacterial and fungal pathogens.[120–124] In addition to the applicability of padlock probes for direct target detection, a universal primer binding site can be introduced into the probe and used for MLPA (see previous discussion).

Microarrays

Applications of microarrays to detect and characterize respiratory viruses began with solid arrays. The first respiratory pan-viral microarray system was described in 2002, which incorporated 1600 unique 70-mer oligonucleotide probes covering approximately 140 viral genome sequences.[60–65] Resequencing microarrays were developed to use short oligonucleotides for the simultaneous identification of respiratory pathogens at both the species and strain level.[125–127] Another comprehensive and panmicrobial microarray, the GreeneChipResp system, was developed for the detection of respiratory viruses and subtype identification of Flu-A viruses.[66] Other recently developed solid microarray systems for detection and identification of a panel of respiratory viruses include the Infiniti analyzer, an integrated molecular diagnostic device incorporating microarray hybridization[128]; the electronic microarray-based Nanochip[85,129]; the TaqMan Low Density Array cards, which use real-time PCR assays for 13 viruses and 8 bacteria known to cause pneumonia (Dean Erdman, 2009; personal communication); and the FilmArray, which detects and differentiates 17 viral and 4 bacterial etiologies of respiratory tract infections (Mark Poritz, 2009; personal communication).

Suspension bead-based liquid xMAP microarrays have been developed by Luminex Corp, which are essentially three-dimensional arrays based on the use of microscopic polystyrene beads as the solid support and flow cytometry for bead and target detection.[130] Robust multiplexing detection is accomplished using different bead sets based on fluorescence. The system enables multiplexing of up to 100 analytes in a single reaction using small sample volumes.[131,132] Numerous studies have described the use of xMAP technology for the detection and differentiation of nucleic acid sequences of microbial pathogens, including enteric bacteria, viruses, mycobacteria, fungi, and protozoa.[76–82,133–136] A molecular typing method incorporating the suspension array was reported to characterize and type Flu-A viruses, including H5N1.[83] The Luminex suspension array has been incorporated into several commercial devices as the detection platform to support the laboratory differential diagnosis of common respiratory viral pathogens. These include the xTAG Respiratory Viral Panel from Luminex Molecular Diagnostics,[137–139] the ResPlex II assay from Qiagen,[78,84,85] and the MultiCode-PLx RVP assay from EraGen Biosciences.[140,141] The suspension array system exhibits rapid hybridization kinetics, flexibility in assay design and format, and relatively low costs, which have made it the most practical microarray platform for clinical diagnostic applications. Users should carefully determine the positive fluorescence threshold for each viral target in multiplexed, user-defined assays during validation.

Mass Spectrometry

Matrix-assisted laser desorption/ionization time-of-flight (MALDI-TOF) mass spectrometry (MS) is widely used as a powerful proteomic tool. Its rapidity and high resolution provide another powerful platform for the detection and characterization of nucleic acid amplification products. The technology is premised on the capacity of MALDI-TOF MS to discriminate individual PCR products contained in complex amplicon mixtures according to nucleotide base composition.[142] The deconvolution algorithm allows base composition of PCR products to be deduced from mass spectrometrically measured molecular weights and the complementary nature of DNA, leading to organism identification. Early studies successfully used this technique to directly detect amplification products from PCR[143] and ligase chain reaction (LCR).[144] Soon after, the MALDI-TOF MS platform was linked to PCR amplification for genotypic analysis of hepatitis C virus[145] and human papillomavirus.[146,147] Detection of human herpesviruses from clinical specimens was performed using MALDI-TOF MS following multiplex PCR amplification.[148] A MALDI-TOF MS-based genotyping assay has been described that monitors development of hepatitis B virus polymerase YMDD mutant genotypes during lamivudine treatment.[149,150]

An integrated system, the Ibis T5000 Biosensor, has been developed to couple broad-range nucleic acid amplification to high-performance electrospray ionization MS and base-composition analysis. The system enables the identification and quantification of a broad set of pathogens, including all known bacteria, all major groups of pathogenic fungi, and the major families of viruses that cause disease in humans and animals, along with the detection of virulence factors and antibiotic resistance markers.[151] The system has been used for rapid identification and strain typing of respiratory bacterial pathogens for epidemic surveillance,[152] identification and genotyping of *Acinetobacter baumannii* strains in an outbreak associated with war trauma,[153,154] determination of quinolone resistance in *Acinetobacter* species,[155,156] genotyping of *Campylobacter* species,[155,156] and rapid genotyping and clonal complex assignment of *Staphylococcus aureus* isolates.[157] We have used this system

Table 1
Comparison of commercially available multiplexed amplification and high-throughput systems for detection and identification of respiratory viruses

System	Company	Viruses/Genotypes Detected	Amplification Platform	Detection Platform	Characteristics
FimArray respiratory pathogen panel	Idaho Technology Inc (Salt Lake City, UT)	AdV, bocavirus, 4 CoV, Flu-A, Flu-B, hMPV, PIV-1, PIV-2, PIV-3, PIV-4, RSV, and RhV	Nested multiplex RT-PCR	Solid array analyzer	Integrated and closed system. Also covers 4 bacterial pathogens
Infiniti respiratory viral panel[128]	AutoGenomics, Inc (Carlsbad, CA)	Flu-A, Flu-B, PIV-1, PIV-2, PIV-3, PIV-4, RSV-A, RSV-B, hMPV-A, hMPV-B, RhV-A, RhV-B, EnV, CoV, and AdV	Multiplex PCR and RT-PCR	Infiniti solid array analyzer	Detection step by the Infiniti analyzer is completely automatic
Jaguar system	HandyLab, Inc (Detroit, MI)	Flu-A, Flu-B, and RSV A/B	Multiplex real-time RT-PCR	Melting temperature analysis	Completely closed and automatic. Universal system compatible with detection of other pathogens. Throughput of 1–24 specimens/run
MultiCode-PLx respiratory virus panel[140,141]	EraGen Biosciences (Madison, WI)	Flu-A, Flu-B, PIV-1, PIV-2, PIV-3, PIV-4, RSV, hMPV, RhV, AdV, and CoV	Multiplex PCR and RT-PCR	Luminex suspension array	Universal beads used for detection use EraCode sequences
NGEN Respiratory Virus (RVA) Analyte-specific reagent[85,129]	Nanogen (San Diego, CA)	Flu-A, Flu-B, PIV-1, PIV-2, PIV-3, and RSV	Multiplex RT-PCR	NanoChip (solid chip)	Discontinued in 2008. Probe labeling, target capture, and detection accomplished using electronic microarray technology

Assay	Company	Targets	Method	Detection	Features
ProFLU+, ProPARAFLU+[161,162]	Prodesse, Inc (Waukesha, WI)	Flu-A, Flu-B, and RSV (ProFLU+); PIV-1, PIV-2, PIV-3, and PIV-4 (ProPARAFLU+)	Multiplex real-time RT-PCR	Melting temperature analysis	ProFLU+ FDA cleared. Limited multiplex formats (triplex)
ResPlex II[78,84,85]	Qiagen (Valencia, CA)	Flu-A, Flu-B, PIV-1, PIV-2, PIV-3, PIV-4, RSV-A, RSV-B, hMPV, RhV, EnV, and SARS-CoV	TEM-RT-PCR	Luminex suspension array	Unique Tem-PCR permits multiple target screening in single reaction without significant loss in sensitivity
Seeplex respiratory virus detection assay[163]	Seegene, Inc (Seoul, Korea)	AdV, hMPV, 2 CoV, PIV-1, PIV-2, PIV-3, Flu-A, Flu-B, RSV-A, RSV-B, and RhV	Two sets of multiplex RT-PCR	Gel electrophoresis	Dual priming oligonucleotide system
xTAG respiratory viral panel (RVP)[137–139]	Luminex Molecular Diagnostics (Toronto, Canada)	Flu-A, Flu-B, PIV-1, PIV-2, PIV-3, PIV-4, RSV-A, RSV-B, hMPV, AdV, EnV, CoV, and RhV	Multiplex PCR and RT-PCR	Luminex suspension array	FDA cleared. Target-specific primer extension used in combination with universal detection beads

Abbreviations: AdV, adenoviruses; CoV, coronaviruses; EnV, enteroviruses; Flu, influenza virus; hMPV, human metapneumovirus; PIV, parainfluenza virus; RhV, rhinoviruses; RSV, respiratory syncytial virus; TEM, target enriched multiplex.

o detect *Ehrlichia*, *Anaplasma*, and *Rickettsia* pathogens directly from blood specimens for diagnosis of tick-borne sepsis (manuscript in preparation). In the field of diagnostic virology, this strategy successfully led to the inclusion of SARS-CoV in the
coronavirus family.[158] Furthermore, the Ibis T5000 Biosensor system has been used
as a rapid and inexpensive tool for global surveillance of emerging Flu virus genotypes[159] and rapid detection and molecular serotyping of adenoviruses.[160] The
system was able to detect and type all available Flu A genotypes, including recently
emerged novel A/H1N1 (David Ecker, 2009; personal communication). The main
advantages are high resolution, speed, and substantial degree of automation. The
main disadvantages include the engineering difficulty of MS device miniaturization
and need for continuous enrichment of databases with new genomic sequences.

MULTIPLEXING AMPLIFICATION AND HIGH-THROUGHPUT DETECTION SYSTEMS

Respiratory infections caused by a many bacterial, viral, and fungal pathogens often
present with overlapping signs and symptoms nearly indistinguishable by clinical diagnosis. Molecular screening of at-risk populations for a group of possible viral pathogens is an exciting area of development in molecular microbiology. Several
multiplexing amplification and high-throughput detection systems are commercially
available for the detection and differentiation of a panel of respiratory viral pathogens.
Examples include the FilmArray platform from Idaho Technology Inc; the Infiniti Respiratory Viral Panel from AutoGenomics, Inc.[128]; the Jaguar system from HandyLab,
Inc.; the Multi-Code-PLx respiratory virus panel from EraGen Biosciences[140,141]; the
NGEN Respiratory Virus ASR from Nanogen[85,129]; the proFLU+ and the proPARA-
FLU+ from Prodesse, Inc.[161,162]; the ResPlex II assay from Qiagen[78,84,85]; the Seeplex
respiratory virus detection assay from Seegene, Inc.[163]; and the xTAG Respiratory
Viral Panel from Luminex Molecular Diagnostics.[137–139] Some of these systems cover
all varieties of Flu A genotypes including recently emerged novel A/H1N1.[164]

A comparative summary of these devices is presented in **Table 1**. Relative
simplicity, powerful multiplexing capabilities, and affordability for high-throughput
detection make these platforms most attractive for screening and detection of a panel
of respiratory viruses in clinical infectious disease diagnostics. Although not essential,
the availability of Food and Drug Administration–cleared products is a critical step in
getting these systems into less-experienced diagnostic microbiology laboratories.[4,5]
Opening of postamplification tubes and subsequent pipetting steps in the workflow
of suspension arrays increases the risk for intra- and inter-run contamination for
some assays. Careful attention should be paid to contamination control measures
and the re-establishment of dedicated postamplification laboratory space in the
real-time PCR era. Simultaneous testing for all possible pathogens is an efficient
means to obtain a conclusive result and improves etiologic diagnosis.[81,137,165] In addition, assaying for all potential pathogens may yield crucial information regarding coinfections or secondary infections.[84,166,167] One study from the Netherlands indicated
that implementation of multiple molecular assays for the etiologic diagnosis of lower
respiratory tract infections increased the diagnostic yield considerably, yet did not
reduce antibiotic use or costs.[168] Clinical relevance and cost effectiveness of simultaneous multipathogen detection and identification strategies merit further investigation.

ACKNOWLEDGMENTS

The authors thank John Brunstein, David Ecker, Dean Erdman, Jiang Fan, and Mark
Poritz for discussion, and James Chappell and Charles Stratton for reviewing the
manuscript.

REFERENCES

1. Ksiazek TG, Erdman D, Goldsmith CS, et al. A novel coronavirus associated with severe acute respiratory syndrome. N Engl J Med 2003;348(20):1953–66.
2. Drosten C, Gunther S, Preiser W, et al. Identification of a novel coronavirus in patients with severe acute respiratory syndrome. N Engl J Med 2003;348(20): 1967–76.
3. Shinde V, Bridges CB, Uyeki TM, et al. Triple-reassortant swine influenza A (H1) in humans in the United States, 2005–2009. N Engl J Med 2009;360(25): 2616–25.
4. Mahony JB. Detection of respiratory viruses by molecular methods. Clin Microbiol Rev 2008;21(4):716–47.
5. Nolte FS. Molecular diagnostics for detection of bacterial and viral pathogens in community-acquired pneumonia. Clin Infect Dis 2008;47(Suppl 3):S123–6.
6. Pejcic B, De Marco R, Parkinson G. The role of biosensors in the detection of emerging infectious diseases. Analyst 2006;131(10):1079–90.
7. Schultz JS. Sensitivity and dynamics of bioreceptor-based biosensors. Ann N Y Acad Sci 1987;506:406–14.
8. Malamud D, Bau H, Niedbala S, et al. Point detection of pathogens in oral samples. Adv Dent Res 2005;18(1):12–6.
9. Zhou X, Liu L, Hu M, et al. Detection of hepatitis B virus by piezoelectric biosensor. J Pharm Biomed Anal 2002;27(1–2):341–5.
10. Ju HX, Ye YK, Zhao JH, et al. Hybridization biosensor using di(2,2′-bipyridine) osmium (III) as electrochemical indicator for detection of polymerase chain reaction product of hepatitis B virus DNA. Anal Biochem 2003;313(2):255–61.
11. Kwakye S, Baeumner A. A microfluidic biosensor based on nucleic acid sequence recognition. Anal Bioanal Chem 2003;376(7):1062–8.
12. Abad-Valle P, Fernandez-Abedul MT, Costa-Garcia A. Genosensor on gold films with enzymatic electrochemical detection of a SARS virus sequence. Biosens Bioelectron 2005;20(11):2251–60.
13. Goldstein AN, Echer CM, Alivisatos AP. Melting in semiconductor nanocrystals. Science 1992;256(5062):1425–7.
14. Michalet X, Pinaud FF, Bentolila LA, et al. Quantum dots for live cells, in vivo imaging, and diagnostics. Science 2005;307(5709):538–44.
15. Edgar R, McKinstry M, Hwang J, et al. High-sensitivity bacterial detection using biotin-tagged phage and quantum-dot nanocomplexes. Proc Natl Acad Sci U S A 2006;103(13):4841–5.
16. Liu WT, Zhu L, Qin QW, et al. Microfluidic device as a new platform for immunofluorescent detection of viruses. Lab Chip 2005;5(11):1327–30.
17. Agrawal A, Tripp RA, Anderson LJ, et al. Real-time detection of virus particles and viral protein expression with two-color nanoparticle probes. J Virol 2005; 79(13):8625–8.
18. Bentzen EL, House F, Utley TJ, et al. Progression of respiratory syncytial virus infection monitored by fluorescent quantum dot probes. Nano Lett 2005;5(4):591–5.
19. Tripp RA, Alvarez R, Anderson B, et al. Bioconjugated nanoparticle detection of respiratory syncytial virus infection. Int J Nanomedicine 2007;2(1):117–24.
20. Lee J, Choi Y, Kim J, et al. Positively charged compact quantum Dot-DNA complexes for detection of nucleic acids. Chemphyschem 2009;10(5):806–11.
21. Chan P, Yuen T, Ruf F, et al. Method for multiplex cellular detection of mRNAs using quantum dot fluorescent in situ hybridization. Nucleic Acids Res 2005; 33(18):e161.

22. Wu X, Liu H, Liu J, et al. Immunofluorescent labeling of cancer marker Her2 and other cellular targets with semiconductor quantum dots. Nat Biotechnol 2003; 21(1):41–6.

23. Notomi T, Okayama H, Masubuchi H, et al. Loop-mediated isothermal amplification of DNA. Nucleic Acids Res 2000;28(12):e63.

24. Mori Y, Nagamine K, Tomita N, et al. Detection of loop-mediated isothermal amplification reaction by turbidity derived from magnesium pyrophosphate formation. Biochem Biophys Res Commun 2001;289(1):150–4.

25. Parida M, Sannarangaiah S, Dash PK, et al. Loop mediated isothermal amplification (LAMP): a new generation of innovative gene amplification technique; perspectives in clinical diagnosis of infectious diseases. Rev Med Virol 2008; 18(6):407–21.

26. Lakshmi V, Neeraja M, Subbalaxmi MV, et al. Clinical features and molecular diagnosis of Chikungunya fever from South India. Clin Infect Dis 2008;46(9): 1436–42.

27. Peyrefitte CN, Boubis L, Coudrier D, et al. Real-time reverse-transcription loop-mediated isothermal amplification for rapid detection of Rift Valley fever virus. J Clin Microbiol 2008;46(11):3653–9.

28. Poon LL, Leung CS, Tashiro M, et al. Rapid detection of the severe acute respiratory syndrome (SARS) coronavirus by a loop-mediated isothermal amplification assay. Clin Chem 2004;50(6):1050–2.

29. Poon LL, Leung CS, Chan KH, et al. Detection of human influenza A viruses by loop-mediated isothermal amplification. J Clin Microbiol 2005;43(1): 427–30.

30. Ito M, Watanabe M, Nakagawa N, et al. Rapid detection and typing of influenza A and B by loop-mediated isothermal amplification: comparison with immunochromatography and virus isolation. J Virol Methods 2006;135(2):272–5.

31. Imai M, Ninomiya A, Minekawa H, et al. Development of H5-RT-LAMP (loop-mediated isothermal amplification) system for rapid diagnosis of H5 avian influenza virus infection. Vaccine 2006;24(44–46):6679–82.

32. Imai M, Ninomiya A, Minekawa H, et al. Rapid diagnosis of H5N1 avian influenza virus infection by newly developed influenza H5 hemagglutinin gene-specific loop-mediated isothermal amplification method. J Virol Methods 2007;141(2): 173–80.

33. Jayawardena S, Cheung CY, Barr I, et al. Loop-mediated isothermal amplification for influenza A (H5N1) virus. Emerg Infect Dis 2007;13(6):899–901.

34. Chen HT, Zhang J, Sun DH, et al. Development of reverse transcription loop-mediated isothermal amplification for rapid detection of H9 avian influenza virus. J Virol Methods 2008;151(2):200–3.

35. Shirato K, Nishimura H, Saijo M, et al. Diagnosis of human respiratory syncytial virus infection using reverse transcription loop-mediated isothermal amplification. J Virol Methods 2007;139(1):78–84.

36. Ushio M, Yui I, Yoshida N, et al. Detection of respiratory syncytial virus genome by subgroups-A, B specific reverse transcription loop-mediated isothermal amplification (RT-LAMP). J Med Virol 2005;77(1):121–7.

37. Hong TC, Mai QL, Cuong DV, et al. Development and evaluation of a novel loop-mediated isothermal amplification method for rapid detection of severe acute respiratory syndrome coronavirus. J Clin Microbiol 2004;42(5):1956–61.

38. Okafuji T, Yoshida N, Fujino M, et al. Rapid diagnostic method for detection of mumps virus genome by loop-mediated isothermal amplification. J Clin Microbiol 2005;43(4):1625–31.

39. Yoshida N, Fujino M, Miyata A, et al. Mumps virus reinfection is not a rare event confirmed by reverse transcription loop-mediated isothermal amplification. J Med Virol 2008;80(3):517–23.
40. Fujino M, Yoshida N, Yamaguchi S, et al. A simple method for the detection of measles virus genome by loop-mediated isothermal amplification (LAMP). J Med Virol 2005;76(3):406–13.
41. Wakabayashi T, Yamashita R, Kakita T, et al. Rapid and sensitive diagnosis of adenoviral keratoconjunctivitis by loop-mediated isothermal amplification (LAMP) method. Curr Eye Res 2004;28(6):445–50.
42. Schouten JP, McElgunn CJ, Waaijer R, et al. Relative quantification of 40 nucleic acid sequences by multiplex ligation-dependent probe amplification. Nucleic Acids Res 2002;30(12):e57.
43. Hsuih TC, Park YN, Zaretsky C, et al. Novel, ligation-dependent PCR assay for detection of hepatitis C in serum. J Clin Microbiol 1996;34(3):501–7.
44. Park YN, Abe K, Li H, et al. Detection of hepatitis C virus RNA using ligation-dependent polymerase chain reaction in formalin-fixed, paraffin-embedded liver tissues. Am J Pathol 1996;149(5):1485–91.
45. Bergval IL, Vijzelaar RN, Dalla Costa ER, et al. Development of multiplex assay for rapid characterization of *Mycobacterium tuberculosis*. J Clin Microbiol 2008; 46(2):689–99.
46. Terefework Z, Pham CL, Prosperi AC, et al. MLPA diagnostics of complex microbial communities: relative quantification of bacterial species in oral biofilms. J Microbiol Methods 2008;75(3):558–65.
47. Reijans M, Dingemans G, Klaassen CH, et al. RespiFinder: a new multiparameter test to differentially identify fifteen respiratory viruses. J Clin Microbiol 2008;46(4):1232–40.
48. Welsh J, McClelland M. Fingerprinting genomes using PCR with arbitrary primers. Nucleic Acids Res 1990;18(24):7213–8.
49. Reyes GR, Kim JP. Sequence-independent, single-primer amplification (SISPA) of complex DNA populations. Mol Cell Probes 1991;5(6):473–81.
50. Williams JG, Kubelik AR, Livak KJ, et al. DNA polymorphisms amplified by arbitrary primers are useful as genetic markers. Nucleic Acids Res 1990;18(22): 6531–5.
51. Power EG. RAPD typing in microbiology—a technical review. J Hosp Infect 1996;34(4):247–65.
52. Winget DM, Wommack KE. Randomly amplified polymorphic DNA PCR as a tool for assessment of marine viral richness. Appl Environ Microbiol 2008;74(9):2612–8.
53. Harcourt BH, Tamin A, Halpin K, et al. Molecular characterization of the polymerase gene and genomic termini of Nipah virus. Virology 2001;287(1): 192–201.
54. Afonso CL. Sequencing of avian influenza virus genomes following random amplification. Biotechniques 2007;43(2):188, 190, 192.
55. Ambrose HE, Clewley JP. Virus discovery by sequence-independent genome amplification. Rev Med Virol 2006;16(6):365–83.
56. Lambden PR, Cooke SJ, Caul EO, et al. Cloning of noncultivatable human rotavirus by single primer amplification. J Virol 1992;66(3):1817–22.
57. Matsui SM, Kim JP, Greenberg HB, et al. The isolation and characterization of a Norwalk virus-specific cDNA. J Clin Invest 1991;87(4):1456–61.
58. Reyes GR, Purdy MA, Kim JP, et al. Isolation of a cDNA from the virus responsible for enterically transmitted non-A, non-B hepatitis. Science 1990; 247(4948):1335–9.

59. van den Hoogen BG, de Jong JC, Groen J, et al. A newly discovered human pneumovirus isolated from young children with respiratory tract disease. Nat Med 2001;7(6):719–24.
60. Wang D, Coscoy L, Zylberberg M, et al. Microarray-based detection and genotyping of viral pathogens. Proc Natl Acad Sci U S A 2002;99(24):15687–92.
61. Wang D, Urisman A, Liu YT, et al. Viral discovery and sequence recovery using DNA microarrays. PLoS Biol 2003;1(2):e2.
62. Chiu CY, Rouskin S, Koshy A, et al. Microarray detection of human parainfluenzavirus 4 infection associated with respiratory failure in an immunocompetent adult. Clin Infect Dis 2006;43(8):e71–6.
63. Urisman A, Molinaro RJ, Fischer N, et al. Identification of a novel Gammaretrovirus in prostate tumors of patients homozygous for R462Q RNASEL variant. PLoS Pathog 2006;2(3):e25.
64. Chiu CY, Alizadeh AA, Rouskin S, et al. Diagnosis of a critical respiratory illness caused by human metapneumovirus by use of a pan-virus microarray. J Clin Microbiol 2007;45(7):2340–3.
65. Chiu CY, Greninger AL, Kanada K, et al. Identification of cardioviruses related to Theiler's murine encephalomyelitis virus in human infections. Proc Natl Acad Sci U S A 2008;105(37):14124–9.
66. Quan PL, Palacios G, Jabado OJ, et al. Detection of respiratory viruses and subtype identification of influenza A viruses by GreeneChipResp oligonucleotide microarray. J Clin Microbiol 2007;45(8):2359–64.
67. Allander T, Andreasson K, Gupta S, et al. Identification of a third human polyomavirus. J Virol 2007;81(8):4130–6.
68. Allander T, Emerson SU, Engle RE, et al. A virus discovery method incorporating DNase treatment and its application to the identification of two bovine parvovirus species. Proc Natl Acad Sci U S A 2001;98(20):11609–14.
69. Allander T, Tammi MT, Eriksson M, et al. Cloning of a human parvovirus by molecular screening of respiratory tract samples. Proc Natl Acad Sci U S A 2005;102(36):12891–6.
70. Djikeng A, Halpin R, Kuzmickas R, et al. Viral genome sequencing by random priming methods. BMC Genomics 2008;9:5.
71. Shi MM. Enabling large-scale pharmacogenetic studies by high-throughput mutation detection and genotyping technologies. Clin Chem 2001;47(2):164–72.
72. van der Hoek L, Pyrc K, Jebbink MF, et al. Identification of a new human coronavirus. Nat Med 2004;10(4):368–73.
73. Braham S, Iturriza-Gomara M, Gray J. Detection of TT virus by single-primer sequence-independent amplification in multiple samples collected from an outbreak of gastroenteritis. Arch Virol 2009;154(6):981–5.
74. Jones MS, Kapoor A, Lukashov VV, et al. New DNA viruses identified in patients with acute viral infection syndrome. J Virol 2005;79(13):8230–6.
75. Jones MS, Lukashov VV, Ganac RD, et al. Discovery of a novel human picornavirus in a stool sample from a pediatric patient presenting with fever of unknown origin. J Clin Microbiol 2007;45(7):2144–50.
76. Han J, Swan DC, Smith SJ, et al. Simultaneous amplification and identification of 25 human papillomavirus types with Templex technology. J Clin Microbiol 2006;44(11):4157–62.
77. Benson R, Tondella ML, Bhatnagar J, et al. Development and evaluation of a novel multiplex PCR technology for molecular differential detection of bacterial respiratory disease pathogens. J Clin Microbiol 2008;46(6):2074–7.

78. Brunstein J, Thomas E. Direct screening of clinical specimens for multiple respiratory pathogens using the Genaco respiratory panels 1 and 2. Diagn Mol Pathol 2006;15(3):169–73.

79. Deng J, Zheng Y, Zhao R, et al. Culture versus polymerase chain reaction for the etiologic diagnosis of community-acquired pneumonia in antibiotic-pretreated pediatric patients. Pediatr Infect Dis J 2009;28(1):53–5.

80. Gegia M, Mdivani N, Mendes RE, et al. Prevalence of and molecular basis for tuberculosis drug resistance in the Republic of Georgia: validation of a QIAplex system for detection of drug resistance-related mutations. Antimicrob Agents Chemother 2008;52(2):725–9.

81. Tang YW, Kilic A, Yang Q, et al. StaphPlex system for rapid and simultaneous identification of antibiotic resistance determinants and Panton-Valentine leukocidin detection of staphylococci from positive blood cultures. J Clin Microbiol 2007;45(6):1867–73.

82. Podzorski RP, Li H, Han J, et al. MVPlex assay for direct detection of methicillin-resistant *Staphylococcus aureus* in Naris and other swab specimens. J Clin Microbiol 2008;46(9):3107–9.

83. Zou S, Han J, Wen L, et al. Human influenza A virus (H5N1) detection by a novel multiplex PCR typing method. J Clin Microbiol 2007;45(6):1889–92.

84. Brunstein JD, Cline CL, McKinney S, et al. Evidence from multiplex molecular assays for complex multipathogen interactions in acute respiratory infections. J Clin Microbiol 2008;46(1):97–102.

85. Li H, McCormac MA, Estes RW, et al. Simultaneous detection and high-throughput identification of a panel of RNA viruses causing respiratory tract infections. J Clin Microbiol 2007;45(7):2105–9.

86. Sanger F, Nicklen S, Coulson AR. DNA sequencing with chain-terminating inhibitors. Proc Natl Acad Sci U S A 1977;74(12):5463–7.

87. Ahmadian A, Ehn M, Hober S. Pyrosequencing: history, biochemistry and future. Clin Chim Acta 2006;363(1–2):83–94.

88. Ronaghi M, Uhlen M, Nyren P. A sequencing method based on real-time pyrophosphate. Science 1998;281(5375):363–5.

89. Borman AM, Linton CJ, Miles SJ, et al. Molecular identification of pathogenic fungi. J Antimicrob Chemother 2008;61(Suppl 1):i7–12.

90. Clarke SC. Pyrosequencing: nucleotide sequencing technology with bacterial genotyping applications. Expert Rev Mol Diagn 2005;5(6):947–53.

91. Tenover FC. Rapid detection and identification of bacterial pathogens using novel molecular technologies: infection control and beyond. Clin Infect Dis 2007;44(3):418–23.

92. Pourmand N, Elahi E, Davis RW, et al. Multiplex pyrosequencing. Nucleic Acids Res 2002;30(7):e31.

93. Costabile M, Quach A, Ferrante A. Molecular approaches in the diagnosis of primary immunodeficiency diseases. Hum Mutat 2006;27(12):1163–73.

94. Lu Y, Boehm J, Nichol L, et al. Multiplex HLA-typing by pyrosequencing. Methods Mol Biol 2009;496:89–114.

95. Pourmand N, Diamond L, Garten R, et al. Rapid and highly informative diagnostic assay for H5N1 influenza viruses. PLoS One 2006;1:e95.

96. Ellis JS, Smith JW, Braham S, et al. Design and validation of an H5 TaqMan real-time one-step reverse transcription-PCR and confirmatory assays for diagnosis and verification of influenza A virus H5 infections in humans. J Clin Microbiol 2007;45(5):1535–43.

97. Duwe S, Schweiger B. A new and rapid genotypic assay for the detection of neuraminidase inhibitor resistant influenza A viruses of subtype H1N1, H3N2, and H5N1. J Virol Methods 2008;153(2):134–41.
98. Bright RA, Medina MJ, Xu X, et al. Incidence of adamantane resistance among influenza A (H3N2) viruses isolated worldwide from 1994 to 2005: a cause for concern. Lancet 2005;366(9492):1175–81.
99. Waybright N, Petrangelo E, Lowary P, et al. Detection of human virulence signatures in H5N1. J Virol Methods 2008;154(1–2):200–5.
100. Bright RA, Shay DK, Shu B, et al. Adamantane resistance among influenza A viruses isolated early during the 2005–2006 influenza season in the United States. JAMA 2006;295(8):891–4.
101. Deyde VM, Nguyen T, Bright RA, et al. Detection of molecular markers of antiviral resistance in influenza A (H5N1) viruses using a pyrosequencing method. Antimicrob Agents Chemother 2009;53(3):1039–47.
102. Deyde VM, Xu X, Bright RA, et al. Surveillance of resistance to adamantanes among influenza A(H3N2) and A(H1N1) viruses isolated worldwide. J Infect Dis 2007;196(2):249–57.
103. Dharan NJ, Gubareva LV, Meyer JJ, et al. Infections with oseltamivir-resistant influenza A(H1N1) virus in the United States. JAMA 2009;301(10):1034–41.
104. Higgins RR, Eshaghi A, Burton L, et al. Differential patterns of amantadine-resistance in influenza A (H3N2) and (H1N1) isolates in Toronto, Canada. J Clin Virol 2009;44(1):91–3.
105. Lackenby A, Democratis J, Siqueira MM, et al. Rapid quantitation of neuraminidase inhibitor drug resistance in influenza virus quasispecies. Antivir Ther 2008;13(6):809–20.
106. Laplante JM, Marshall SA, Shudt M, et al. Influenza antiviral resistance testing in New York and Wisconsin, 2006 to 2008: methodology and surveillance data. J Clin Microbiol 2009;47(5):1372–8.
107. Elahi E, Pourmand N, Chaung R, et al. Determination of hepatitis C virus genotype by pyrosequencing. J Virol Methods 2003;109(2):171–6.
108. Gharizadeh B, Kalantari M, Garcia CA, et al. Typing of human papillomavirus by pyrosequencing. Lab Invest 2001;81(5):673–9.
109. Kramski M, Meisel H, Klempa B, et al. Detection and typing of human pathogenic hantaviruses by real-time reverse transcription-PCR and pyrosequencing. Clin Chem 2007;53(11):1899–905.
110. O'Meara D, Wilbe K, Leitner T, et al. Monitoring resistance to human immunodeficiency virus type 1 protease inhibitors by pyrosequencing. J Clin Microbiol 2001;39(2):464–73.
111. Rajeevan MS, Swan DC, Duncan K, et al. Quantitation of site-specific HPV 16 DNA methylation by pyrosequencing. J Virol Methods 2006;138(1–2):170–6.
112. Trama JP, Adelson ME, Mordechai E. Identification and genotyping of molluscum contagiosum virus from genital swab samples by real-time PCR and pyrosequencing. J Clin Virol 2007;40(4):325–9.
113. Hoper D, Hoffmann B, Beer M. Simple, sensitive, and swift sequencing of complete H5N1 avian influenza virus genomes. J Clin Microbiol 2009;47(3):674–9.
114. Nilsson M, Malmgren H, Samiotaki M, et al. Padlock probes: circularizing oligonucleotides for localized DNA detection. Science 1994;265(5181):2085–8.
115. Landegren U, Nilsson M. Locked on target: strategies for future gene diagnostics. Ann Med 1997;29(6):585–90.

116. Szemes M, Bonants P, de Weerdt M, et al. Diagnostic application of padlock probes—multiplex detection of plant pathogens using universal microarrays. Nucleic Acids Res 2005;33(8):e70.
117. van Doorn R, Szemes M, Bonants P, et al. Quantitative multiplex detection of plant pathogens using a novel ligation probe-based system coupled with universal, high-throughput real-time PCR on OpenArrays. BMC Genomics 2007;8:276.
118. Gyarmati P, Conze T, Zohari S, et al. Simultaneous genotyping of all hemagglutinin and neuraminidase subtypes of avian influenza viruses by use of padlock probes. J Clin Microbiol 2008;46(5):1747–51.
119. Baner J, Gyarmati P, Yacoub A, et al. Microarray-based molecular detection of foot-and-mouth disease, vesicular stomatitis and swine vesicular disease viruses, using padlock probes. J Virol Methods. 2007;143(2):200–6.
120. Kaocharoen S, Wang B, Tsui KM, et al. Hyperbranched rolling circle amplification as a rapid and sensitive method for species identification within the *Cryptococcus* species complex. Electrophoresis 2008;29(15):3183–91.
121. Kong F, Tong Z, Chen X, et al. Rapid identification and differentiation of *Trichophyton* species, based on sequence polymorphisms of the ribosomal internal transcribed spacer regions, by rolling-circle amplification. J Clin Microbiol 2008;46(4):1192–9.
122. Tong Z, Kong F, Wang B, et al. A practical method for subtyping of Streptococcus agalactiae serotype III, of human origin, using rolling circle amplification. J Microbiol Methods 2007;70(1):39–44.
123. van Doorn R, Slawiak M, Szemes M, et al. Robust detection and identification of multiple oomycetes and fungi in environmental samples using a novel cleavable padlock probe-based ligation-detection assay. Appl Environ Microbiol 2009;75(12):4185–93.
124. Wamsley HL, Barbet AF. In situ detection of Anaplasma spp. by DNA target-primed rolling-circle amplification of a padlock probe and intracellular colocalization with immunofluorescently labeled host cell von Willebrand factor. J Clin Microbiol 2008;46(7):2314–9.
125. Lin B, Blaney KM, Malanoski AP, et al. Using a resequencing microarray as a multiple respiratory pathogen detection assay. J Clin Microbiol 2007;45(2):443–52.
126. Malanoski AP, Lin B, Wang Z, et al. Automated identification of multiple microorganisms from resequencing DNA microarrays. Nucleic Acids Res 2006;34(18):5300–11.
127. Wang Z, Daum LT, Vora GJ, et al. Identifying influenza viruses with resequencing microarrays. Emerg Infect Dis 2006;12(4):638–46.
128. Raymond F, Carbonneau J, Boucher N, et al. Comparison of automated microarray detection with real-time PCR assays for detection of respiratory viruses in specimens obtained from children. J Clin Microbiol 2009;47(3):743–50.
129. Takahashi H, Norman SA, Mather EL, et al. Evaluation of the NanoChip 400 system for detection of influenza A and B, respiratory syncytial, and parainfluenza viruses. J Clin Microbiol 2008;46(5):1724–7.
130. Horan PK, Wheeless LL Jr. Quantitative single cell analysis and sorting. Science 1977;198(4313):149–57.
131. Armstrong B, Stewart M, Mazumder A. Suspension arrays for high throughput, multiplexed single nucleotide polymorphism genotyping. Cytometry 2000;40(2):102–8.

32. Dunbar SA, Vander Zee CA, Oliver KG, et al. Quantitative, multiplexed detection of bacterial pathogens: DNA and protein applications of the Luminex LabMAP system. J Microbiol Methods 2003;53(2):245–52.

33. Dunbar SA, Jacobson JW. Quantitative, multiplexed detection of *Salmonella* and other pathogens by Luminex xMAP suspension array. Methods Mol Biol 2007; 394:1–19.

34. McNamara DT, Thomson JM, Kasehagen LJ, et al. Development of a multiplex PCR-ligase detection reaction assay for diagnosis of infection by the four parasite species causing malaria in humans. J Clin Microbiol 2004;42(6):2403–10.

35. Schmitt M, Bravo IG, Snijders PJ, et al. Bead-based multiplex genotyping of human papillomaviruses. J Clin Microbiol 2006;44(2):504–12.

36. Tarr CL, Patel JS, Puhr ND, et al. Identification of *Vibrio* isolates by a multiplex PCR assay and rpoB sequence determination. J Clin Microbiol 2007;45(1): 134–40.

137. Mahony J, Chong S, Merante F, et al. Development of a respiratory virus panel test for detection of twenty human respiratory viruses by use of multiplex PCR and a fluid microbead-based assay. J Clin Microbiol 2007;45(9):2965–70.

138. Merante F, Yaghoubian S, Janeczko R. Principles of the xTAG respiratory viral panel assay (RVP Assay). J Clin Virol 2007;40(Suppl 1):s31–5.

139. Pabbaraju K, Tokaryk KL, Wong S, et al. Comparison of the Luminex xTAG respiratory viral panel with in-house nucleic acid amplification tests for diagnosis of respiratory virus infections. J Clin Microbiol 2008;46(9):3056–62.

140. Lee WM, Grindle K, Pappas T, et al. High-throughput, sensitive, and accurate multiplex PCR-microsphere flow cytometry system for large-scale comprehensive detection of respiratory viruses. J Clin Microbiol 2007;45(8):2626–34.

141. Nolte FS, Marshall DJ, Rasberry C, et al. MultiCode-PLx system for multiplexed detection of seventeen respiratory viruses. J Clin Microbiol 2007; 45(9):2779–86.

142. Muddiman DC, Anderson GA, Hofstadler SA, et al. Length and base composition of PCR-amplified nucleic acids using mass measurements from electrospray ionization mass spectrometry. Anal Chem 1997;69(8):1543–9.

143. Hurst GB, Doktycz MJ, Vass AA, et al. Detection of bacterial DNA polymerase chain reaction products by matrix-assisted laser desorption/ionization mass spectrometry. Rapid Commun Mass Spectrom 1996;10(3):377–82.

144. Jurinke C, van den Boom D, Jacob A, et al. Analysis of ligase chain reaction products via matrix-assisted laser desorption/ionization time-of-flight-mass spectrometry. Anal Biochem 1996;237(2):174–81.

145. Kim YJ, Kim SO, Chung HJ, et al. Population genotyping of hepatitis C virus by matrix-assisted laser desorption/ionization time-of-flight mass spectrometry analysis of short DNA fragments. Clin Chem 2005;51(7):1123–31.

146. Hong SP, Shin SK, Lee EH, et al. High-resolution human papillomavirus genotyping by MALDI-TOF mass spectrometry. Nat Protoc 2008;3(9):1476–84.

147. Soderlund-Strand A, Dillner J, Carlson J. High-throughput genotyping of oncogenic human papilloma viruses with MALDI-TOF mass spectrometry. Clin Chem 2008;54(1):86–92.

148. Sjoholm MI, Dillner J, Carlson J. Multiplex detection of human herpesviruses from archival specimens by using matrix-assisted laser desorption ionization-time of flight mass spectrometry. J Clin Microbiol 2008;46(2):540–5.

149. Hong SP, Kim NK, Hwang SG, et al. Detection of hepatitis B virus YMDD variants using mass spectrometric analysis of oligonucleotide fragments. J Hepatol 2004;40(5):837–44.

150. Lee CH, Kim SO, Byun KS, et al. Predominance of hepatitis B virus YMDD mutants is prognostic of viral DNA breakthrough. Gastroenterology 2006 130(4):1144–52.
151. Ecker DJ, Sampath R, Massire C, et al. Ibis T5000: a universal biosensor approach for microbiology. Nat Rev Microbiol 2008;6(7):553–8.
152. Ecker DJ, Sampath R, Blyn LB, et al. Rapid identification and strain-typing of respiratory pathogens for epidemic surveillance. Proc Natl Acad Sci U S A 2005;102(22):8012–7.
153. Ecker JA, Massire C, Hall TA, et al. Identification of Acinetobacter species and genotyping of *Acinetobacter baumannii* by multilocus PCR and mass spectrometry. J Clin Microbiol 2006;44(8):2921–32.
154. Wortmann G, Weintrob A, Barber M, et al. Genotypic evolution of *Acinetobacter baumannii* strains in an outbreak associated with war trauma. Infect Control Hosp Epidemiol 2008;29(6):553–5.
155. Hannis JC, Manalili SM, Hall TA, et al. High-resolution genotyping of *Campylobacter* species by use of PCR and high-throughput mass spectrometry. J Clin Microbiol 2008;46(4):1220–5.
156. Hujer KM, Hujer AM, Endimiani A, et al. Rapid determination of quinolone resistance in *Acinetobacter* spp. J Clin Microbiol 2009;47(5):1436–42.
157. Hall TA, Sampath R, Blyn LB, et al. Rapid molecular genotyping and clonal complex assignment of *Staphylococcus aureus* isolates by PCR/ESI-MS. J Clin Microbiol 2009;47(6):1733–61.
158. Sampath R, Hofstadler SA, Blyn LB, et al. Rapid identification of emerging pathogens: coronavirus. Emerg Infect Dis 2005;11(3):373–9.
159. Sampath R, Russell KL, Massire C, et al. Global surveillance of emerging Influenza virus genotypes by mass spectrometry. PLoS One 2007;2(5):e489.
160. Blyn LB, Hall TA, Libby B, et al. Rapid detection and molecular serotyping of adenovirus by use of PCR followed by electrospray ionization mass spectrometry. J Clin Microbiol 2008;46(2):644–51.
161. Legoff J, Kara R, Moulin F, et al. Evaluation of the one-step multiplex real-time reverse transcription-PCR ProFlu-1 assay for detection of influenza A and influenza B viruses and respiratory syncytial viruses in children. J Clin Microbiol 2008;46(2):789–91.
162. Liao RS, Tomalty LL, Majury A, et al. Comparison of viral isolation and multiplex real-time reverse transcription-PCR for confirmation of respiratory syncytial virus and influenza virus detection by antigen immunoassays. J Clin Microbiol 2009; 47(3):527–32.
163. Kim SR, Ki CS, Lee NY. Rapid detection and identification of 12 respiratory viruses using a dual priming oligonucleotide system-based multiplex PCR assay. J Virol Methods 2009;156(1–2):111–6.
164. Ginocchio CC, St George K. Likelihood that an unsubtypeable influenza A result in the Luminex xTAG respiratory virus panel is indicative of novel A/H1N1 (swine-like) influenza. J Clin Microbiol 2009;47(7):2347–8.
165. Templeton KE, Scheltinga SA, van den Eeden WC, et al. Improved diagnosis of the etiology of community-acquired pneumonia with real-time polymerase chain reaction. Clin Infect Dis 2005;41(3):345–51.
166. Chung JY, Han TH, Kim SW, et al. Respiratory picornavirus infections in Korean children with lower respiratory tract infections. Scand J Infect Dis 2007;39(3): 250–4.

167. Pierangeli A, Gentile M, Di Marco P, et al. Detection and typing by molecular techniques of respiratory viruses in children hospitalized for acute respiratory infection in Rome, Italy. J Med Virol 2007;79(4):463–8.
168. Oosterheert JJ, van Loon AM, Schuurman R, et al. Impact of rapid detection of viral and atypical bacterial pathogens by real-time polymerase chain reaction for patients with lower respiratory tract infection. Clin Infect Dis 2005;41(10): 1438–44.

The Human Bocaviruses: A Review and Discussion of Their Role in Infection

Brian D.W. Chow, MD[a,b,c], Frank P. Esper, MD[a,b,d],*

KEYWORDS

• Human bocavirus • Human bocavirus 2 • Human bocavirus 3
• Viral infection • Viral gastroenteritis • Pneumonia

Respiratory tract infections are a major cause of morbidity and mortality. Lower respiratory tract disease accounts for approximately 4 million deaths annually worldwide. Of all hospital discharges in the United States, close to 10% are attributed to diseases of the respiratory system with an estimated mortality of 232,000 in 2005.[1] The economic burden of these infections in the United States is projected to be more than $100 billion.[2]

Viruses, such as influenza, respiratory syncytial virus (RSV), and parainfluenza viruses, are known to be responsible for most respiratory tract infections. In a significant proportion of respiratory tract disease, however, no pathogen is identified. Over the last 10 years, the advancement of molecular detection and genomic amplification has led to the recognition of numerous potential respiratory pathogens, including the human metapneumovirus (HMPV),[3] human coronaviruses NL63,[4–6] HKU1,[7] and SARS-CoV,[8] Ki and WU polyomaviruses,[9,10] and the human bocavirus (HBoV).[11] Although disease caused by respiratory viruses has been underestimated in the past, there is now a growing appreciation for the role these viruses play in community- and hospital-acquired pneumonia.

The HBoV is a novel parvovirus first isolated in 2005 from human respiratory secretions from patients who had pneumonia.[11] Since that time, it has been

a Case Western Reserve University, 10900 Euclid Avenue, Cleveland, OH 44106, USA
b Department of Pediatrics, University Hospitals Case Medical Center, 11100 Euclid Avenue, Cleveland, OH 44106, USA
c Department of Internal Medicine, University Hospitals Case Medical Center, 11100 Euclid Avenue, Cleveland, OH 44106, USA
d Division of Pediatric Infectious Diseases, Rainbow Babies and Children's Hospital, 11100 Euclid Avenue, Cleveland, OH 44106, USA
* Corresponding author. Division of Pediatric Infectious Diseases, Rainbow Babies and Children's Hospital, 11100 Euclid Avenue, Cleveland, OH 44106.
E-mail address: frank.esper@uhhospitals.org (F.P. Esper).

Clin Lab Med 29 (2009) 695–713
doi:10.1016/j.cll.2009.07.010
0272-2712/09/$ – see front matter © 2009 Elsevier Inc. All rights reserved.

labmed.theclinics.com

associated with upper and lower respiratory tract disease and gastrointestinal illness in adult and pediatric patients throughout the world. Recently, two viruses closely related to the human bocavirus have been reported, provisionally named human bocavirus 2 (HboV-2) and human bocavirus 3 (HBoV-3).[12,13] For the sake of clarity the remainder of this article refers to the original human bocavirus strain described by Allander and colleagues as human bocavirus 1 (HBoV-1).[11] It remains unclear whether HBoV-1, HBoV-2, and HBoV-3 represent unique viral entities or distant genotypes of a single virus. Because HBoV-2 and HBoV-3 have only been recognized over the last several months, the epidemiology and clinical manifestations associated with these viruses are only now being realized. The incidence of human bocaviruses varies widely,[14,15] with various clinical presentations, and they are often found in association with other potential pathogens. This phenomenon has led to debate over the role of human bocaviruses as true pathogens. This article reviews the published studies and discusses the virologic, clinical, and diagnostic aspects of these newly recognized human viruses.

DISCOVERY OF HUMAN BOCAVIRUSES
Human Bocavirus 1

HBoV-1 was first described by Allander and colleagues[11] in 2005. Pooled, cell-free supernatant from respiratory samples was examined using a random polymerase chain reaction (PCR) technique. Amplified PCR products were separated, ligated to a vector, and introduced into *Escherichia coli*. Clones were sequenced and evaluated through an automated protocol and compared against known sequences. The majority of the clones were determined to be human or recognized bacterial and viral pathogens. Of the remaining sequences, a parvoviruslike sequence was identified with no known correlation to recognized human parvoviruses. Phylogenetic analysis showed this to be a novel parvovirus most closely related to bovine parvovirus and canine minute virus (**Fig. 1**). It is now named the human bocavirus.

Human Bocavirus 2

In January 2009, Kapoor and colleagues[12] reported the identification of a related parvovirus, termed HBoV-2, from pediatric stool samples by random PCR analysis of nuclease-resistant virus particles. The resulting amplicons were subcloned into a plasmid vector, sequenced, and compared with genome entries on GenBank. Phylogenetic analysis of HBoV-2 shows that it is most closely related to HBoV-1. The amino acid identity of HBoV-2 to HBoV-1 is 78%, 67%, and 80% for the NS1, NP1, and VP1/VP2 proteins, respectively. There is significant divergence of the genomic targets used for detection of HBoV-1, which explains why HBoV-2 has remained unidentified to this point.

Human Bocavirus 3

A third bocavirus species was described in April 2009 from Australia, and has been provisionally named human bocavirus 3 (HBoV-3). Similar to the methods used in discovery of HBoV-1 and HBoV-2, Arthur and colleagues[13] digested filtered fecal samples with nucleases, then pelleted virions and evaluated using degenerate oligonucleotide primed–PCR. During these investigations, the group simultaneously discovered HBoV-2 and a third species of bocavirus, HBoV-3. Analysis of the genome shows close homology to HBoV-1 in the nonstructural protein encoding regions (NS1, NP1), but HBoV-3 is more similar to HBoV-2 in the structural protein encoding regions (VP1/VP2). This finding suggests that HBoV3 may be the product

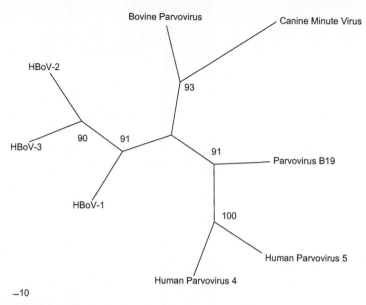

Fig. 1. Phylogenetic analysis of Animal and Human Parvovirus Species. Unrooted radial tree of representative animal and human parvovirus strains (HBoV-1 [GenBank accession no. NC_007455.1], HBoV-2 [NC_012042.1]; HBoV-3 [NC_012564.1]; Bovine Parvovirus [DQ335247.1], Canine Minute Virus [NC_004442.1], Parvovirus B19 [AY386330.1]; Human Parvovirus 4 [EU874248.1], and Human Parvovirus 5 [DQ873391.1]) is displayed. Maximum-likelihood phylogenetic trees were constructed using the PHYLIP program DNAML, with the default transition to transversion ratio of 2.0 and 1 jumble. One hundred bootstrap data sets were created using the PHYLIP program SEQBOOT. Bootstrap values are displayed at major branch points.

of recombination between HBoV1 and HBoV2. Arthur and colleagues identified a recombination site that supports this hypothesis. As with HBov-2, the HBoV-3 genome is divergent enough from HBoV-1 to explain lack of detection using currently published primer sets (**Table 1**). Clinical presentation, seasonal distribution, and prevalence of HBoV3 have yet to be characterized in full. Further analysis of the phylogenetic relationships will be required to determine the correct taxonomy of this virus family.

BIOLOGY AND TAXONOMY

Human bocaviruses are parvoviruses belonging to the family Parvoviridae, subfamily Parvovirinae, and are most closely related to bovine parvovirus and canine minute virus, in the genus *Betaparvovirus* (see **Fig. 1**). Parvoviruses are single-stranded DNA viruses with a small genome size between 4 kilobases (kb) and 6 kb that have three open reading frames that encode two nonstructural proteins, NS1 and NP1, and the structural VP1 and VP2 proteins. The HBoV genome does not encode a polymerase and depends on host cell DNA polymerases for replication. Parvoviruses have unenveloped capsids with icosahedral symmetry.[16] Based on electron micrographs, HBoV-1 appears structurally similar to other members of the Parvoviridae family and is approximately 25 nm in diameter.[17]

Table 1

Nucleic acid amplification methods and primer sets used for detection of human bocavirus 1

		Target Gene	Target Location[a]	Predicted Size (bp)	Forward Primer	Reverse Primer	Probe[b]	% Detected[c] (Median[d])	References
Polymerase chain reaction	Conventional	NP1	2351-2704	353	GACCTCTGTAAGTCTATTAC	CTCTGTTGACTGAATACAG		0.8-45.2 (5.4)	11,14,20,24,28,29,34,38-40, 47,48,62-75,83,102
		NS1	2301-2700	399	CCCAAGAAACGTGTCTAAC	GTGTTGACTGAATACAGTGT		2.8-2.9 (2.90)	62,63,76,103-105
		VP1/VP2	1545-1835	290	TATGGCCAAGGCAATCGTCCAAG	GCCGGCGTGAAACATGAGAAACAGA		0.8-11.3 (5.5)	35,40-43,49,56,59,60,77,102
		VP1/VP2	4125-4966	841	GTGACCACCAAGTACTTAGAACTGG	GCTCTCTCCCAGTGACAT		5.1-12.5 (8.8)	24,47,66,74
		VP1/VP2	4370-5189	819	GGACCACAGTCATCAGAC	CCACTACCATCGGGCTG		3.5-5.5% (4.50)	42,43
		VP1/VP2	3639-4286	647	TTCAGAATGGTCACCTCTACA	CTGTGCTTCCGTTTTGTCTTA		6.60	65
		VP1/VP2	4562-4966	404	GCAAACCCATCACTCTCAATGC	GCTCTCTCTCCCAGTAGACAT		1.5-14.2 (7.6)	14,24,47,66,74
		VP1/VP2	4268-4467	199	AGACAAAACGGAAGCACAGC	TCAAAGCCAGATCCAAATCC		3.10	84
		VP1/VP2	4269-4467	198	CAGTGGTACCAGACACCAGAAG	GCCAGTTCTTTGTGCGTATCT		5.5-31.3 (14.0)	25,84
		VP1/VP2	4270-4467	197	CCAAAAAGAGACACTTTTACTTTGCTAACTCA	TGGACGCCAGTTCTTTGTTGCGTATCTTTC		2.2-2.7 (2.40)	48
	Nested	NP1	2259-3259	1000	Outer: GAAGACACCGAGCCTGAGAC	Outer: GCTGATTGGGTTGTTCCTGAT		7.10	106
			2351-2565	214	Inner: GAGCTCTGTAAGTCTATTAC	Inner: ATATGAGCCCGAGCCTCT			
	Paired Nested[e]	NP1	2318-2709	391	Outer: TAAACTGCTCCAGCAAGTCCTCCA	Outer: GGAAGCTCTGTTGACTGAAT		7.4-11.1 (9.3)	107,108
			2344-2709	365	Inner: CTCACCTGCGAGCCTGTAAGTA	Inner: GGAAGCTCTGTTGACTGAAT			
		VP1/VP2	4085-4988	903	Outer: GCACTTCTGTATCAGATGCCTT	Outer: CGTGGTATGTAGGCCGTGTAG			
			4139-4988	849	Inner: CTTAGAACTGGTGGAGCACTG	Inner: CGTTGGTATGTAGGCGTGTAG			
		NS1	1579-1794	215	Outer: TATGGGTGTGTTAATCATTTGAAYA	Outer: GTAGATATCGTGRTTRGTKGATAT		5.80	50
			1600-1703	103	Inner: AACAAAGGATTTGTWTYAAYGAYTG	Inner: CCCAAGATACACTTTGCWKGTTCCACCC			
		NS1	2325-2723	398	Outer: CCAGCAAGTCCCAAACTACCTGC	Outer: GGAGCTTCAGGATTGGAAGCTCTGTG			
			2351-2704	353	Inner: GAGCTCTGTAAGTCTATTAC	Inner: CTCTGTTGACTGAATACAG			

Method	Target	Location	Primer/Probe 1	Primer/Probe 2	Primer/Probe 3	Range of % (median)	References
Real-time	NP1	22548–2628, 2570	AGAGGCTCGGGCTCATATCA	CACTTGGTCTTGAGGTCTTCGAA	AGGAACACCCAATCARCCACCTAtGtCt	2.9–32.3 (9.1)	21,28,??
	NP1	2509–2605, 2534	AGGAGCAGGAGCCGCAGCC	CAGTGCAAGACGATAGGTGGC	ATGAGCCGGAGCCTCTCCCCACTGTGTC	9	22
	NP1	2397–2592, 2533	CCACGTGACGAAGATGAGCTC	TAGGTGGCTGATTGGGTGTTC	CCGAGCCTCTCTCCCCACTGTGTCG	11.9	78
	NP1	2405–2586, 2506	CGAAGAATGAGCTCAGGGAAT	GCTGATTGGGTGTTCCTGAT	CACAGGAGCAGGAGCCGCAG	9.0–11.3 (10.7)	17,51,67,86
	NP1	2427–2580, 2504	GAAAGACAAGCATCGCTCC	TGGGGTGTTCCTGATGATATG	CGCGCTGGAGCAGGAGCCGCAGCCCGATAGGCG	2.9	87
	NP1	2351–2704, 2480	GAGCTCTGTAAGTACTATTAC	CTCTGTGTTGACTGAATACAG	GGAAGAGACATGGCAGACAAC	12.8	79
	NP1	2391–2466, 2411	GCACAGCCACGTGGCAGACAA	TGGACTCCCTTTCTTTTTGTAGGA	TGAGCTCAGGGAATATGAAAGACAAGCATCGTMR	4.6	44
	NP1	2480–2579, 2504	GGAAGAGACACTGGCAGACAA	GGGGTGTTCCTGCTCCTGATATGAGC	CTGCGGCCTCCTGCTCCTGTGAT	2.4–18.9 (5.3)	15,26,30,88
	NP1	2424–2636, 2559	TATGAAAGACAAGCATCGCTCCTA	GTCTTCATCACTTGGTCTGAGGTCT	CTCATATCATCAGGAACAC	8.2	37
	NP1	2554–2628, 2577	TCGGGCTCATATCATCAGGAA	CACTTGGTCTGAGGTCTTCGAA	CCCAATCAGCCACCTATCGTTGC	19.3	83
	NP1	2488–2566, 2512	CACTGGCAGACAACTCATCACA	GATATGAGCCCGAGCCTCT	AGCAGGAGCCCGCAGCCCGA	4.5	89
	NP1	1617–1710, 1667	TAATGACTGGCAGACAACGCCTAG	TGTCCCGCCAAGATACACT	TTCCACCCAATCCTGGT	9	90
	NP1	1637–1711, 1668	TAGTTGTTTGGTGGGARGA	CTGTCCCGCCAAGATACA	CCAGGATTGGGTGGAACCTGCAAA	9.1	54
	NP1	1624–1711, 1668	TGCAGAACAACGCYTAGTTGTTT	CTGTCCCGCCAAGATACA	CCAGGATTGGGTGGAACCTGCAAA	2.9–32.3 (3.5)	36,42,85
NASBA[f]	NP1	2567–2424, 2456	AATTCTAATAGCGACTRCACTATA-GGGGCTGATTGGGTGTCCTGAT	AATTCTAATAGACTACTAATAGGGC-GAAGATGAGCTCAGGGAAT	CGATCGAGTCGAGAAAGA-GGGGAGGAGCGGATCG	0	94

[a] Estimated location based on GenBank isolate EU262978.1, probe location added when applicable.

[b] Added when applicable.

[c] Range of percent detected in cited studies.

[d] Median of percent detected in cited studies when applicable.

[e] In cited studies, a sample positive for HBoV-1 required amplification from both sets of nested PCR primers.

[f] Nucleic acid sequence based amplification.

[g] Case reports.

The VP2 gene is nested in the reading frame of VP1 and uses an alternate initiator codon.[11] The sequence of VP1 and VP2 differ only in the N-terminal extension of VP1. This region, referred to as the VP1 unique region, plays a critical role in virus infectivity in some parvoviruses.[18] In several parvoviruses, VP3 arises from posttranslational proteolytic cleavage of VP2 proteins. It remains unclear if VP3 exists in human bocavirus. The capsid of parvoviruses consists of about 60 copies of each viral capsid protein. The role of NS1 and NP1 proteins in human bocavirus species remain unknown. Zhi and colleagues[19] created an infectious clone of the related parvovirus B19 to determine the functions of these genes. Their findings showed that NS and VP1 knockout mutants abolished the viral infectivity. The NS protein also seemed to be vital in genome transcription and to play a role in the regulation of capsid gene expression.

Parvoviruses have been shown to be transmitted by various routes, including respiratory, urine, and fecal–oral contact.[16] The mode of bocavirus transmission of HBoV is unknown. Most studies have reported the presence of HBoV-1 DNA in respiratory secretions and fecal samples. HBoV-1 DNA has also been detected in addition to serum, urine, and lymph nodes.[20–22] So far, HBoV-2 and HBoV-3 have only been identified in stool samples. Similar to other respiratory viruses, transmission may occur through several routes, including inhalation, contact with infected secretions (through direct contact or possibly contaminated surfaces), and fecal–oral from the standpoint of gastrointestinal illness.

Although some parvoviruses cannot replicate without helper viruses, the mechanisms of cell entry and replication have not been described for human bocavirus. This lack of information is largely because of the inability to grow human bocaviruses in standard cell lines.

CLINICAL PRESENTATION
Bocaviruses and Respiratory Illness

Following Allander's initial description of HBoV-1 in the human respiratory tract[11], more than 60 studies have been published investigating the role of this virus in respiratory tract illness. Clinical findings reported from HBoV-1–positive patients from 9 representative studies are summarized in **Table 2**. Most patients present with symptoms of upper respiratory tract illness, including cough, fever, and rhinorrhea. Pharyngitis and rash are less common (11%–13%). Additionally, patients tended to report earache.[14,23]

Several studies raise the possibility that HBoV-1 is associated with severe respiratory disease. Reports describe this virus in children hospitalized for bronchiolitis,[24] asthma exacerbations,[15,25] and first-time episodes of wheezing.[26] Wheezing is described in numerous studies. In one prospective study comparing 16 respiratory viruses in children admitted with respiratory infection, wheezing was seen in more than 50% of children in whom HBoV-1 was recognized as the sole agent. Surprisingly, children who had coinfections had less wheezing.[27] Other common findings include tachypnea, fever, and hypoxia. One report from Jordan found as many of 18% of children hospitalized with pneumonia were positive for HBoV-1.[28] In Thailand, Fry and colleagues found that patients who had HBoV-1 were more likely to be hospitalized with pneumonia (odds ratio of 3.56) compared with controls.

Most HBoV-1 reports are retrospective analyses based from hospital settings In these studies, up to 6.6% of patients required stays in intensive care units and up to 40% required oxygen therapy at some point during their hospitalization.[20,29] These studies likely overestimate the severity of disease associated with HBoV-1 because of selection bias. In studies based on community samples, disease is mild and only rarely requires admission. To date, there have been no reported deaths associated with HBoV-1.

Few studies list underlying comorbidities in HBoV-1–infected patients. When reported, more than half of patients had an underlying medical condition.[20] The most common underlying conditions involve primary cardiac or pulmonary disease, including congenital heart lesions, heart failure, asthma, chronic obstructive pulmonary disease, and prematurity with chronic lung disease.[11,20,29]

HBoV-1 has been reported in immunocompromised patients who have respiratory and gastrointestinal illness. Schenk and colleagues[22] reported a child coinfected with rhinovirus and HBoV-1 following hematopoietic stem cell transplant. This patient developed fever, dyspnea, wheezing, and infiltrates on chest radiograph. In this patient, HBoV-1 DNA was isolated from nasopharyngeal, stool, and blood samples. Koskenvuo and colleagues[30] reported a series of children who had acute lymphoblastic leukemia in whom HBoV-1 was identified. Presenting symptoms were febrile upper respiratory infection with otitis media, fever with vomiting and diarrhea, and isolated fever. Garbino and colleagues[31] reported a case of HBoV-1 in a hospitalized adult infected with HIV. All patients eventually recovered from their acute illness.

Although few studies have systematically examined immunocompromised patients for HBoV-1, the incidence seems to be low. One study by Muller and colleagues[32] examined bronchoalveolar lavage specimens from immunocompromised patients suspected of having *Pneumocystis jiroveci* pneumonia. Only 1 specimen of 128 (0.8%) was found to have HBoV-1. Miyakis and colleagues[33] prospectively examined bronchoalveolar lavage specimens from 53 adult lung transplant recipients and 67 symptomatic nontransplant patients and failed to find HBoV-1 in any sample. These studies argue against HBoV-1 as a pathogen of lower respiratory tract disease in these vulnerable populations.

Because many of these reports observe high coinfection rates, it is difficult to draw conclusions as to whether HBoV-1 plays a role in pathogenicity of infected patients. To answer this several studies have compared the presence of HBoV-1 in asymptomatic control groups to symptomatic individuals.[34–37] All but one found HBoV-1 more often in symptomatic children than in healthy controls. In the remaining study, asymptomatic carriage of HBoV-1 was as frequent in asymptomatic infants as those who had acute respiratory tract disease. In a recent report by Allander and colleagues[15] HBoV-1 DNA is also present in the serum of acutely ill patients suggesting that dissemination of this virus is possible. These findings provide support for HBoV-1 as a cause for respiratory illness. When in vitro culture systems and animal models are available, a better understanding of the role of HBoV-1 in human respiratory disease can be established.

Bocaviruses and Gastrointestinal Symptoms

Gastrointestinal symptoms are reported in up to 25% of patients who have HBoV-1 respiratory infection (see **Table 2**) suggesting HBoV-1 may not be limited to the respiratory tract alone. The closely related canine and bovine parvoviruses are well described as both respiratory and enteric pathogens.[16] Subsequent investigations have identified HBoV-1 DNA in stool samples from patients with gastrointestinal illness. The most common gastrointestinal symptoms include nausea, vomiting, and diarrhea. Both watery and bloody diarrhea have been reported in conjunction with HBoV-1.[38–45]

HBoV-1 has been identified in 0.8% to 9.1% of stool samples from patients presenting with gastrointestinal illness.[38–43] HBoV-1 viral load in stool is significantly less than viral loads found in respiratory tract specimens of symptomatic patients.[44] Similar to studies of respiratory illness, HBoV-1 is commonly codetected with recognized enteric pathogens, with coinfection rates ranging from 21% to 77.6%.[41,43] Identified copathogens include norovirus, rotavirus, human calicivirus, astrovirus, adenovirus, Campylobacter, Salmonella, and Clostridium difficile.[38–40,42–44] In a recent case-control study on acute gastroenteritis, Arthur and colleagues[13] examined stool specimens for potential pathogens, including all three species of human bocavirus. DNA from human bocaviruses 1, 2, or 3 was isolated from 54 (27.4%) stool samples, making these human bocaviruses the second most common viral agents identified after rotavirus (37.1%). Clinical illness associated with HBoV-1 and rotavirus coinfection did not seem to be significantly different than that of rotavirus illness alone, suggesting the presence of HBoV-1 did not worsen disease.[42]

HBoV-1 is infrequently reported in stools originating from immunocompromised patients. In a 4-year-old patient who had diarrhea, bocavirus was recognized on day 21 and again on day 75 following stem cell transplant. This patient went on to develop disseminated disease.[22] One patient who had a T cell deficiency was reported to have hepatitis associated with HBoV-1.[46] HBoV-1 was also associated with gastroenteritis in one patient who had B cell immunodeficiency.[39] Unlike HBoV-1–associated respiratory disease, large investigations for HBoV-1–associated gastrointestinal illness have not been performed for the immunocompromised population.

As with respiratory disease, the role of HBoV-1 as a cause for gastrointestinal disease is unclear. Several reports have identified HBoV-1 in stool samples from asymptomatic patients.[42,44] Arthur and colleagues compared stool samples positive for HBoV-1, HBoV-2, and HBoV-3 from symptomatic patients and age-matched asymptomatic controls. The presence of HBoV-1 failed to achieve statistical significance, supporting the hypothesis that HBoV-1 may not be a cause of acute gastroenteritis.[13] The authors note that the lack of HBoV-1 in symptomatic individuals may be because symptoms may appear before viral particles are shed in stool. Similar findings were made for astrovirus and adenovirus, which are widely accepted causes of gastroenteritis.[13] Also, HBoV-2 was significantly found more often in patients with gastroenteritis. Because of the low incidence in this study, the clinical significance of HBoV-3 remains unclear. Further data on higher viral load in stool samples corresponding with active disease would support causality.

HUMAN BOCAVIRUS 1 COINFECTIONS

Most studies identify coinfecting viral and bacterial pathogens in a substantial percentage of HBoV-1–positive samples. Although all studies did not examine samples for all pathogens, commonly reported pathogens include enterovirus, rhinovirus, RSV, parainfluenza, influenza, adenovirus, and HMPV (**Table 3**).

HBoV-1 coinfection was a common occurrence in all studies with a median rate of 42.5%. HBoV-1 coinfection is described with numerous pathogens; however, those that screen positive for rhinovirus, enteroviruses, and influenza have the highest incidence of HBoV-1 coinfection. Similarly, in samples found positive for HBoV-1, a high rate of enterovirus, influenza, and RSV is seen. Although this likely reflects the high frequency of these viruses in the population at large, one may speculate that these particular coinfecting viruses may provide a biologic benefit to HBoV.

EPIDEMIOLOGY OF HUMAN BOCAVIRUSES

HBoV-1 has been recognized worldwide in association with upper and lower respiratory disease. Most HBoV-1–positive samples originate from children predominantly

ounger than 2 years of age.[11,20,27,29,34–36,47–53] Within this age group, children less
nan 6 months of age seem to be less frequently affected, perhaps because of passive
naternal immunity. Several studies have detected HBoV-1 in adults.[20,54,55] In one
tudy screening 1539 children and 273 adults, HBoV-1 occurred at a similar frequency
n both groups.[20]

Seasonal Distribution

Most studies report circulation of HBoV-1 predominantly during the winter
season.[20,47] Seasonal peaks vary but most often are described in the early winter.
Most of these studies are retrospective, using archived respiratory samples submitted
or analysis of common respiratory pathogens. This approach may lead to misrepre-
sentation of when this virus circulates. Several reports show increased frequency of
HBoV-1 infections during the spring. Choi and colleagues[56] screened samples over
a 5-year period from patients who had lower respiratory tract illness (LRTI) in Korea
and found a higher frequency of HBoV-1 between May and July. Bastien and
colleagues[14] studied samples originating from patients in Canada and reported no
apparent seasonal prevalence. Only a few prospective studies of HBoV-1 have
been performed. In a 1-year prospective investigation in children less than 5 years
of age hospitalized with respiratory tract disease, HBoV-1 was detected in every
month except August.[51] In this study HBoV-1 peaked in the month of December,
with 80% of HBoV-1 isolates occurring between November and March.

Seroepidemiology

Several seroepidemiology studies have been performed to assess the prevalence of
HBoV-1 infection during childhood. Kahn and colleagues reported anti–HBoV-1 antibodies are common in children.[57] Screening serum samples using a viruslike particle–
based ELISA, Kahn and colleagues found evidence of prior HBoV-1 infection in 195 of
270 (72.2%) serum samples.[57] Children between 4 and 8 months of age had the
lowest prevalence of antibodies against HBoV-1, whereas children younger than 2
months of age and those older than 5 years had the highest.[57,58] The high proportion
of seropositive children younger than 2 months of age suggests vertical transfer of
antibodies. The subsequent decline in the percentage of seropositive children over
the first 4 to 6 months of life likely represents waning maternal immunity. The low
percentage of anti-HBoV antibodies in children younger than 12 months of age correlates with population-based studies that demonstrate children younger than 1 year of
age have a higher occurrence of infection.[20,29,34] By 5 years of age, most people have
circulating antibodies against HBoV-1, similar to other respiratory viruses, such as
RSV,[59] rhinovirus,[60] and HMPV.[61]

Because of the difficulties of growing HBoV-1 in vitro, it has yet to be determined
which antibodies offer protection. Also it is unclear if antibodies against HBoV-1 will
confer protection against HBoV-2 or HBoV-3 and vice versa. Most protective antibodies are speculated to target the two viral capsid proteins VP1 and VP2. HBoV-2
and HBoV-3 both have approximately 80% AA identity with HBoV-1 in this region
with most sequence diversion occurring in the N terminal portion. The high similarity
of viral capsid proteins suggest cross-reactive antibodies between bocavirus species
may occur. Studies on HBoV-2 and HBoV-3 seroepidemiology have not been
performed thus far and are warranted.

Sequence Analysis of Bocavirus Species

As more bocavirus species are recognized, our understanding of this family of viruses
grows. Based on the available sequence data of HBoV-1, there seem to be two closely

Table 2
Clinical findings of patients positive for human bocavirus 1

N[a]	Respiratory Findings									GI Findings			References
	Cough	Fever	Rhinorrhea	O$_2$ Therapy	Hypoxia	Tachypnea	Wheeze	Pharyngitis	Other Respiratory Symptoms[b]	Nausea or Vomiting	Diarrhea	Other GI Symptoms[c]	
32	26	18	22	10	10	11	10	—	1	8	5	0	38
68	58	42	46	30	28	—	—	—	59	21	14	—	65d
14	—	10	—	—	7	11	—	—	14	0	0	0	11
30	23	13	27	—	—	6	6	—	—	6	7	—	73
9	9	9	0	5	—	2	2	—	—	—	—	—	70
95	81	75	72	—	—	—	—	11	24	28	7	11	26d
18	12	12	6	—	—	—	—	7	—	2	—	—	14d
32	28	21	28	12	—	—	—	—	26	4	5	—	49d
33	13	—	9	12	—	—	10	1	23	—	—	3	42
Total[e]	250	200	210	69	45	30	28	19	147	69	38	14	—
No. evaluated[f]	317	298	317	174	14	85	104	146	304	289	271	174	—
Occurrence (%)	78.9	67.1	66.2	39.7	39.5	35.3	26.9	13.0	48.4	23.9	14.0	8.0	—

Abbreviation: GI, gastrointestinal.

[a] Number evaluated in each study.
[b] Includes respiratory distress, increased work of breathing, cyanosis, apnea, rhonchi, rales, shortness of breath.
[c] Includes abdominal pain, poor feeding, unspecified GI complaints.
[d] Clinical analysis includes patients who have respiratory copathogens identified in addition to HBoV-1.
[e] Cumulative patients reported with listed findings.
[f] Cumulative patients evaluated for listed finding.

related genotypes. The two prototype strains (ST1, DQ000495.1; ST2, NC_007455.1) have 99.5% identity at the nucleotide and protein level. Because the amino acid identity between both genotypes differs by so little, it may be assumed they represent one serotype. Analysis of 24 HBoV-1 unique isolates (12 originating from respiratory samples and 12 from fecal samples) demonstrated little sequence variation from the prototypic strains.[39] There was also no difference in the proportion of each HBoV-1 genotype identified in nasopharyngeal and fecal isolates, suggesting that each lineage infects both respiratory and enteric systems.

The recent recognition of HBoV-2 and HBoV-3 demonstrates that the bocavirus genus has substantial diversity. HBoV-2 and HBoV-3 have similar genomic organization of the putative open reading frames (ORFs) to HBoV-1. Phylogenetic analysis of HBoV-2 ORFs show that it is more closely related to HBoV-1 (pairwise distance 22.2%–26.2%) than to the animal bocaviruses (pairwise distance 46.2%–55.8%).[12] HBoV-3 nonstructural proteins NS1 and NP1 are closely related to HBoV-1, whereas the structural viral capsid proteins are more similar to HBoV-2 (see **Fig. 1**). Arthur and colleagues[13] hypothesize that HBoV-3 may be a result of a distant recombination event between HBoV-1 and HBoV-2. Because only several strains of HBoV-2 and HBoV-3 have been recognized from a handful of regions worldwide, however, the true diversity is unclear.

DETECTION OF HUMAN BOCAVIRUSES
Polymerase Chain Reaction

Following the discovery of human bocavirus, numerous studies have used conventional PCR to detect HBoV-1.[14,20,24,28,29,34,35,38–41,43,48,49,56,58,60,62–82] Primers, target genes, and predicted amplicon sizes are listed in **Table 1**. Most primer sets used for HBoV-1 screening target the NP1 gene. Although there is a wide variation in detection of HBoV-1 between study sites with detection rates as high as 45.2% reported in one study,[72] primers targeting the VP1/VP2 region have a slightly higher detection rate (median 7.5%, see **Table 1**). This difference is not surprising because the VP1/VP2 is more conserved than NS or NP. In addition, nested and real-time PCR have been used to detect HBoV-1. Real-time PCR yields a slightly higher median frequency of detection of HBoV-1.[15,17,21,26,30,36,37,44,51,52,54,67,68,83–93] The variation in detection of HBoV-1 in these studies is likely attributable to multiple factors, including sensitivity of primer sets, laboratory technique, true variation in incidence of HBoV-1, and methods used in sample collection.

Ziegler and colleagues[94] reported using nucleic acid sequence based amplification (NASBA) to screen for HBoV-1 in stool samples. NASBA is an isothermic nucleic acid amplification technique used as an alternative to PCR for the detection of viruses.[95,96] In the study by Ziegler and coworkers,[94] no HBoV-1 was detected using NASBA. It is unclear if this represents a failure of the method, lack of HBoV-1 in the samples, reaction inhibitors to stool samples, or other variables.

An increasing number of studies are screening stool samples for the presence of HBoV-1.[38,39,41–44] Based on fecal and respiratory HBoV sequence similarities reported by Lau and colleagues genomic targets used for respiratory samples should be as successful in stool samples.[39] The current literature finds that HBoV-1 is found in stool samples less often than in respiratory samples (median 2% versus 7.5%). It is unclear whether this lower rate of detection is due to a truly lower incidence of HBoV-1 in stool, decreased viral loads, or presence of reaction inhibitors commonly found in feces.

Cell Culture and Animal Models

To date, HBoV-1 has not been successfully propagated in standard cell lines or animal models. This failure has been one of the major impediments to our understanding of this virus. Parvoviruses have a large host range and tissue tropism, even among closely related strains. The viral capsid proteins seem to be the major determinant of host specificity.[16] The related human parvovirus B19 causes viremia and replicates in the bone marrow of children and adults and in the liver of the fetus.[16] Two studies identified HBoV-1 DNA in serum of affected patients. Fry and colleagues[36] demonstrated HBoV-1 in acute serum from HBoV-1–positive children who had respiratory disease. Allander and colleagues[15] detected HBoV-1 DNA in more than half of acute-phase serum samples and in 19% of the convalescent-phase serum specimens. Detection of HBoV-1 in serum was associated with a high viral load in the nasopharynx. Even with the detection of HBoV-1 DNA in the blood of affected patients, however, it remains unclear if HBoV-1 viremia truly occurs.

THERAPY

Among healthy children, viral respiratory disease is often a self-limited and uncomplicated disease. Therapy against most viral respiratory pathogens has not been shown to be effective. Treatment of viral pathogens, such as influenza, may shorten the duration of illness in low-risk patients but has not been shown to reduce the duration of illness in the high-risk population.[97] Treatment with ribavirin or intravenous immune globulin (IVIG) remain controversial in the setting of viral respiratory disease and are only used in select populations with severe RSV and human parainfluenza virus (HPIV) disease.[98,99]

The relative ineffectiveness of antiviral compounds is, in part, because host inflammatory reaction leads to a substantial amount of pathology. In addition, many patients present for medical attention at a time past peak viral replication. For these reasons, it is difficult to demonstrate effectiveness of most antiviral compounds.

In several case reports, patients have received antiviral treatment either as prophylaxis or as treatment of confirmed or presumed viral infections. Schenck and colleagues[22] reported a child who had undergone hematopoietic stem cell transplant who was receiving acyclovir prophylaxis; however, he subsequently developed symptomatic HBoV-1 disease with HBoV-1 DNA identified in respiratory, blood, and stool samples. During this patient's complicated hospital course, he was placed on ganciclovir and eventually foscarnet for cytomegalovirus (CMV) viremia. Both the CMV viral load and the HBoV-1 serum viral load became undetectable after initiating foscarnet. This patient continued to have HBoV-1 DNA detectable in stool samples, however. Kupfer and colleagues[100] reported a patient undergoing treatment of B-cell lymphoma who received ganciclovir for CMV viremia who was also found to have HBoV-1 in respiratory secretions. There was no clinical improvement in symptoms after initiating ganciclovir.

Supportive care, even in the intensive care setting, plays a large role in the management of patients who have severe viral illness. Supplemental oxygen[22] and mechanical ventilation[101] have been used to support patients who have HBoV-1–associated disease. In one study, up to 28% of HBoV-1–positive children required intensive care, although not all required respiratory assistance.[20] One patient, coinfected with RSV and HBoV-1, required support through extracorporeal membrane oxygenation until underlying cardiac physiology could be repaired.

There have been no comparative studies using antiviral agents for the treatment of human bocaviruses. The large percentage of coinfections associated with human

Table 3
Human bocavirus 1 detection and coinfection in relation to common respiratory viruses

	RSV (%)	Influenza[d](%)	PIV[e](%)	HMPV (%)	Rhinovirus (%)	Enterovirus (%)	Coronaviruses[f] (%)
Frequency of HBoV-1[a]	1.6–31.3 (7.1)	1.6–31.2 (9.8)	1.6–31.3 (8.0)	1.7–19.3 (7.7)	1.6–19.3 (7.7)	2.4–19.3 (12.5)	1.7–19.3 (7.8)
Bocavirus 1 samples with copathogen[b]	15.0	9.0	3.8	5.6	8.0	13.0%	0.0
Listed virus-positive samples coinfected with HBoV-1[c]	6.5	10.3	6.5	5.9	9.5	13.45	0.0

Abbreviations: HMPV, human metapneumovirus; HBoV-1, human bocavirus 1; RSV, respiratory syncytial virus; PIV, parainfluenza virus.
[a] Frequency (median) of human bocavirus 1 in studies that also screened for listed virus.
[b] Median number of human bocavirus 1–positive samples found to be coinfected with listed pathogen.
[c] Median number of samples positive for listed virus found to be coinfected with human bocavirus 1.
[d] Includes pooled results for Influenza A, B, and C. Not all studies included all members.
[e] Includes types 1–4. Not all studies included all members.
[f] Includes 229E, OC43, HKU1, and NL 63. Not all studies included all members.

bocavirus infections suggests that evaluation for further pathogens should be undertaken for any patient diagnosed with HBoV-1. Treatment of copathogens (ie, influenza, may lead to patient improvement. Future therapeutic strategies may include vaccines, HBoV-neutralizing antibodies, and small interfering RNA.

DISCUSSION

Three human bocavirus species are now recognized and are reported in association with respiratory and gastrointestinal diseases. Because of wide variation in clinical presentations, severity of disease, and a high rate of coinfection, the role of the bocaviruses in causing disease has been debated. One consideration is that bocaviruses are passenger viruses with little or no clinical effect. Another possibility is that bocaviruses require the presence of a copathogen for infection. Several studies suggest that this is not the case, however. Bocavirus is identified in patients who have disease despite the absence of copathogens. Case-control studies have shown an increased risk for pneumonia in patients who have HBoV-1–positive respiratory secretions and increased risk for gastroenteritis in patients who have HBoV-2–positive fecal samples. Two studies found no increase in HBoV-1 frequency in symptomatic versus asymptomatic stool samples. One report finds HBoV-1 did not worsen gastrointestinal disease when coinfected with known pathogens such as rotavirus.[13] The question of whether HBoV-2 or HBoV-3 is associated with respiratory infection has not been answered.

Little is known about the recently described bocaviruses HBoV-2 and HBoV-3. Clinical epidemiology and seroepidemiology have yet to be described in detail. Although antibodies to HBoV-1 are common in human sera, cross-reactivity with HBoV-2 and HBoV-3 has not been investigated. Furthermore, although HBoV-2 and HBoV-3 have been described in stool, their presence in the respiratory tract should be investigated.

Areas for further research on HBoV-1 include examining objective measures of disease severity in patients who have coinfections and examining HBoV-1 for evidence of disease distant to the respiratory and gastrointestinal tracts. Presence of HBoV-1 has been described in serum,[22] lymphatic tissue,[21] and in conjunction with elevated hepatic enzymes,[46] the clinical significance of which has yet to be determined.

In summary, although the evidence for pathogenicity of human bocaviruses is increasing, more research is needed to determine severity of HBoV-associated disease and clinical outcomes.

REFERENCES

1. Merrill C, Elixhauser A. Hospitalization in the United States, 2002: HCUP fact book no. 6. Rockville (MD): Agency for Healthcare Research and Quality; 2005.
2. Birnbaum HG, Morley M, Greenberg PE, et al. Economic burden of respiratory infections in an employed population. Chest 2002;122(2):603–11.
3. van den Hoogen BG, de Jong JC, Groen J, et al. A newly discovered human pneumovirus isolated from young children with respiratory tract disease. Nat Med 2001;7(6):719–24.
4. van der Hoek L, Pyrc K, Jebbink MF, et al. Identification of a new human coronavirus. Nat Med 2004;10(4):368–73.
5. Fouchier RA, Hartwig NG, Bestebroer TM, et al. A previously undescribed coronavirus associated with respiratory disease in humans. Proc Natl Acad Sci U S A 2004;101(16):6212–6.

6. Esper F, Weibel C, Ferguson D, et al. Evidence of a novel human coronavirus that is associated with respiratory tract disease in infants and young children. J Infect Dis 2005;191(4):492–8.
7. Woo PC, Lau SK, Chu CM, et al. Characterization and complete genome sequence of a novel coronavirus, coronavirus HKU1, from patients with pneumonia. J Virol 2005;79(2):884–95.
8. Drosten C, Gunther S, Preiser W, et al. Identification of a novel coronavirus in patients with severe acute respiratory syndrome. N Engl J Med 2003;348(20): 1967–76.
9. Allander T, Andreasson K, Gupta S, et al. Identification of a third human polyomavirus. J Virol 2007;81(8):4130–6.
10. Gaynor AM, Nissen MD, Whiley DM, et al. Identification of a novel polyomavirus from patients with acute respiratory tract infections. PLoS Pathog 2007;3(5):e64.
11. Allander T, Tammi MT, Eriksson M, et al. Cloning of a human parvovirus by molecular screening of respiratory tract samples. Proc Natl Acad Sci U S A 2005;102(36):12891–6.
12. Kapoor A, Slikas E, Simmonds P, et al. A newly identified bocavirus species in human stool. J Infect Dis 2009;199(2):196–200.
13. Arthur JL, Higgins GD, Davidson GP, et al. A novel bocavirus associated with acute gastroenteritis in Australian children. PLoS Pathog 2009;5(4):e1000391.
14. Bastien N, Brandt K, Dust K, et al. Human bocavirus infection, Canada. Emerg Infect Dis 2006;12(5):848–50.
15. Allander T, Jartti T, Gupta S, et al. Human bocavirus and acute wheezing in children. Clin Infect Dis 2007;44(7):904–10.
16. Burns K, Parrish CR. Parvoviridae. In: Fields BN, Knipe DM, Howley PM, editors. Fields' virology. 5th edition. Philadelphia: Wolters Kluwer Health/Lippincott Williams & Wilkins; 2007. p. 2437–66.
17. Brieu N, Gay B, Segondy M, et al. Electron microscopy observation of human bocavirus (HBoV) in nasopharyngeal samples from HBoV-infected children. J Clin Microbiol 2007;45(10):3419–20.
18. Lindner J, Modrow S. Human bocavirus—a novel parvovirus to infect humans. Intervirology 2008;51(2):116–22.
19. Zhi N, Mills IP, Lu J, et al. Molecular and functional analyses of a human parvovirus B19 infectious clone demonstrates essential roles for NS1, VP1, and the 11-kilodalton protein in virus replication and infectivity. J Virol 2006;80(12):5941–50.
20. Chow BD, Huang YT, Esper FP. Evidence of human bocavirus circulating in children and adults, Cleveland, Ohio. J Clin Virol 2008;43(3):302–6.
21. Lu X, Gooding LR, Erdman DD. Human bocavirus in tonsillar lymphocytes. Emerg Infect Dis 2008;14(8):1332–4.
22. Schenk T, Strahm B, Kontny U, et al. Disseminated bocavirus infection after stem cell transplant. Emerg Infect Dis 2007;13(9):1425–7.
23. Monteny M, Niesters HG, Moll HA, et al. Human bocavirus in febrile children, The Netherlands. Emerg Infect Dis 2007;13(1):180–2.
24. Jacques J, Moret H, Renois F, et al. Human bocavirus quantitative DNA detection in French children hospitalized for acute bronchiolitis. J Clin Virol 2008;43(2):142–7.
25. Gendrel D, Guedj R, Pons-Catalano C, et al. Human bocavirus in children with acute asthma. Clin Infect Dis 2007;45(3):404–5.
26. Bosis S, Esposito S, Niesters HG, et al. Role of respiratory pathogens in infants hospitalized for a first episode of wheezing and their impact on recurrences. Clin Microbiol Infect 2008;14(7):677–84.

27. Garcia ML, Calvo C, Pozo F, et al. Detection of human bocavirus in ill and healthy Spanish children: a 2-year study. Arch Dis Child 2009;94(3):249.
28. Kaplan NM, Dove W, Abu-Zeid AF, et al. Human bocavirus infection among children, Jordan. Emerg Infect Dis 2006;12(9):1418–20.
29. Arnold JC, Singh KK, Spector SA, et al. Human bocavirus: prevalence and clinical spectrum at a children's hospital. Clin Infect Dis 2006;43(3):283–8.
30. Koskenvuo M, Mottonen M, Waris M, et al. Human bocavirus in children with acute lymphoblastic leukemia. Eur J Pediatr 2008;167(9):1011–5.
31. Garbino J, Inoubli S, Mossdorf E, et al. Respiratory viruses in HIV-infected patients with suspected respiratory opportunistic infection. AIDS 2008;22(6):701–5.
32. Muller A, Klinkenberg D, Vehreschild J, et al. Low prevalence of human metapneumovirus and human bocavirus in adult immunocompromised high risk patients suspected to suffer from Pneumocystis pneumonia. J Infect 2009; 58(3):227–31.
33. Miyakis S, van Hal SJ, Barratt J, et al. Absence of human Bocavirus in bronchoalveolar lavage fluid of lung transplant patients. J Clin Virol 2009; 44(2):179–80.
34. Kesebir D, Vazquez M, Weibel C, et al. Human bocavirus infection in young children in the United States: molecular epidemiological profile and clinical characteristics of a newly emerging respiratory virus. J Infect Dis 2006;194(9):1276–82.
35. Maggi F, Andreoli E, Pifferi M, et al. Human bocavirus in Italian patients with respiratory diseases. J Clin Virol 2007;38(4):321–5.
36. Fry AM, Lu X, Chittaganpitch M, et al. Human bocavirus: a novel parvovirus epidemiologically associated with pneumonia requiring hospitalization in Thailand. J Infect Dis 2007;195(7):1038–45.
37. von Linstow ML, Hogh M, Hogh B. Clinical and epidemiologic characteristics of human bocavirus in Danish infants: results from a prospective birth cohort study. Pediatr Infect Dis J 2008;27(10):897–902.
38. Chieochansin T, Thongmee C, Vimolket L, et al. Human bocavirus infection in children with acute gastroenteritis and healthy controls. Jpn J Infect Dis 2008; 61(6):479–81.
39. Lau SK, Yip CC, Que TL, et al. Clinical and molecular epidemiology of human bocavirus in respiratory and fecal samples from children in Hong Kong. J Infect Dis 2007;196(7):986–93.
40. Lee JI, Chung JY, Han TH, et al. Detection of human bocavirus in children hospitalized because of acute gastroenteritis. J Infect Dis 2007;196(7):994–7.
41. Albuquerque MC, Rocha LN, Benati FJ, et al. Human bocavirus infection in children with gastroenteritis, Brazil. Emerg Infect Dis 2007;13(11):1756–8.
42. Cheng WX, Jin Y, Duan ZJ, et al. Human bocavirus in children hospitalized for acute gastroenteritis: a case-control study. Clin Infect Dis 2008;47(2):161–7.
43. Yu JM, Li DD, Xu ZQ, et al. Human bocavirus infection in children hospitalized with acute gastroenteritis in China. J Clin Virol 2008;42(3):280–5.
44. Campe H, Hartberger C, Sing A. Role of Human Bocavirus infections in outbreaks of gastroenteritis. J Clin Virol 2008;43(3):340–2.
45. Schildgen O, Muller A, Simon A. Human bocavirus and gastroenteritis. Emerg Infect Dis 2007;13(10):1620–1.
46. Kainulainen L, Waris M, Soderlund-Venermo M, et al. Hepatitis and human bocavirus primary infection in a child with T-cell deficiency. J Clin Microbiol 2008; 46(12):4104–5.
47. Bastien N, Chui N, Robinson JL, et al. Detection of human bocavirus in Canadian children in a 1-year study. J Clin Microbiol 2007;45(2):610–3.

48. Canducci F, Debiaggi M, Sampaolo M, et al. Two-year prospective study of single infections and co-infections by respiratory syncytial virus and viruses identified recently in infants with acute respiratory disease. J Med Virol 2008; 80(4):716–23.
49. Chung JY, Han TH, Kim CK, et al. Bocavirus infection in hospitalized children, South Korea. Emerg Infect Dis 2006;12(8):1254–6.
50. Manning A, Russell V, Eastick K, et al. Epidemiological profile and clinical associations of human bocavirus and other human parvoviruses. J Infect Dis 2006; 194(9):1283–90.
51. Brieu N, Guyon G, Rodiere M, et al. Human bocavirus infection in children with respiratory tract disease. Pediatr Infect Dis J 2008;27(11):969–73.
52. Catalano-Pons C, Bue M, Laude H, et al. Human bocavirus infection in hospitalized children during winter. Pediatr Infect Dis J 2007;26(10):959–60.
53. Garcia-Garcia ML, Calvo C, Pozo F, et al. Human bocavirus detection in nasopharyngeal aspirates of children without clinical symptoms of respiratory infection. Pediatr Infect Dis J 2008;27(4):358–60.
54. Longtin J, Bastien M, Gilca R, et al. Human bocavirus infections in hospitalized children and adults. Emerg Infect Dis 2008;14(2):217–21.
55. Zheng MQ, Lin F, Zheng MY, et al. [Clinical prospective study on maternal-fetal transmission of human bocavirus]. Zhonghua Shi Yan He Lin Chuang Bing Du Xue Za Zhi 2007;21(4):331–3.
56. Choi EH, Lee HJ, Kim SJ, et al. The association of newly identified respiratory viruses with lower respiratory tract infections in Korean children, 2000–2005. Clin Infect Dis 2006;43(5):585–92.
57. Kahn JS, Kesebir D, Cotmore SF, et al. Seroepidemiology of human bocavirus defined using recombinant virus-like particles. J Infect Dis 2008;198(1):41–50.
58. Endo R, Ishiguro N, Kikuta H, et al. Seroepidemiology of human bocavirus in Hokkaido prefecture, Japan. J Clin Microbiol 2007;45(10):3218–23.
59. Gilchrist S, Torok TJ, Gary HE Jr, et al. National surveillance for respiratory syncytial virus, United States, 1985–1990. J Infect Dis 1994;170(4):986–90.
60. Arden KE, McErlean P, Nissen MD, et al. Frequent detection of human rhinoviruses, paramyxoviruses, coronaviruses, and bocavirus during acute respiratory tract infections. J Med Virol 2006;78(9):1232–40.
61. Esper F, Martinello RA, Boucher D, et al. A 1-year experience with human metapneumovirus in children aged <5 years. J Infect Dis 2004;189(8):1388–96.
62. Simon A, Groneck P, Kupfer B, et al. Detection of bocavirus DNA in nasopharyngeal aspirates of a child with bronchiolitis. J Infect 2007;54(3):e125–7.
63. Volz S, Schildgen O, Klinkenberg D, et al. Prospective study of Human Bocavirus (HBoV) infection in a pediatric university hospital in Germany 2005/2006. J Clin Virol 2007;40(3):229–35.
64. Chieochansin T, Chutinimitkul S, Payungporn S, et al. Complete coding sequences and phylogenetic analysis of Human Bocavirus (HBoV). Virus Res 2007;129(1):54–7.
65. Chieochansin T, Samransamruajkit R, Chutinimitkul S, et al. Human bocavirus (HBoV) in Thailand: clinical manifestations in a hospitalized pediatric patient and molecular virus characterization. J Infect 2008;56(2):137–42.
66. Cilla G, Onate E, Perez-Yarza EG, et al. Viruses in community-acquired pneumonia in children aged less than 3 years old: High rate of viral coinfection. J Med Virol 2008;80(10):1843–9.
67. Foulongne V, Olejnik Y, Perez V, et al. Human bocavirus in French children. Emerg Infect Dis 2006;12(8):1251–3.

68. Foulongne V, Rodiere M, Segondy M. Human Bocavirus in children. Emerg Infect Dis 2006;12(5):862–3.
69. IP M, Nelson EA, Cheuk ES, et al. Pediatric hospitalization of acute respiratory tract infections with Human Bocavirus in Hong Kong. J Clin Virol 2008;42(1):72–4.
70. Ma X, Endo R, Ishiguro N, et al. Detection of human bocavirus in Japanese children with lower respiratory tract infections. J Clin Microbiol 2006;44(3):1132–4.
71. Naghipour M, Cuevas LE, Bakhshinejad T, et al. Human bocavirus in Iranian children with acute respiratory infections. J Med Virol 2007;79(5):539–43.
72. Neske F, Blessing K, Tollmann F, et al. Real-time PCR for diagnosis of human bocavirus infections and phylogenetic analysis. J Clin Microbiol 2007;45(7):2116–22.
73. Redshaw N, Wood C, Rich F, et al. Human bocavirus in infants, New Zealand. Emerg Infect Dis 2007;13(11):1797–9.
74. Vicente D, Cilla G, Montes M, et al. Human bocavirus, a respiratory and enteric virus. Emerg Infect Dis 2007;13(4):636–7.
75. Weissbrich B, Neske F, Schubert J, et al. Frequent detection of bocavirus DNA in German children with respiratory tract infections. BMC Infect Dis 2006;6:109.
76. Terrosi C, Fabbiani M, Cellesi C, et al. Human bocavirus detection in an atopic child affected by pneumonia associated with wheezing. J Clin Virol 2007;40(1):43–5.
77. Zhang LL, Tang LY, Xie ZD, et al. Human bocavirus in children suffering from acute lower respiratory tract infection in Beijing Children's Hospital. Chin Med J (Engl) 2008;121(17):1607–10.
78. Christensen A, Nordbo SA, Krokstad S, et al. Human bocavirus commonly involved in multiple viral airway infections. J Clin Virol 2008;41(1):34–7.
79. Kleines M, Scheithauer S, Rackowitz A, et al. High prevalence of human bocavirus detected in young children with severe acute lower respiratory tract disease by use of a standard PCR protocol and a novel real-time PCR protocol. J Clin Microbiol 2007;45(3):1032–4.
80. Chung JY, Han TH, Kim SW, et al. Detection of viruses identified recently in children with acute wheezing. J Med Virol 2007;79(8):1238–43.
81. Sloots TP, McErlean P, Speicher DJ, et al. Evidence of human coronavirus HKU1 and human bocavirus in Australian children. J Clin Virol 2006;35(1):99–102.
82. Tan BH, Lim EA, Seah SG, et al. The incidence of human bocavirus infection among children admitted to hospital in Singapore. J Med Virol 2009;81(1):82–9.
83. Bonzel L, Tenenbaum T, Schroten H, et al. Frequent detection of viral coinfection in children hospitalized with acute respiratory tract infection using a real-time polymerase chain reaction. Pediatr Infect Dis J 2008;27(7):589–94.
84. Catalano-Pons C, Giraud C, Rozenberg F, et al. Detection of human bocavirus in children with Kawasaki disease. Clin Microbiol Infect 2007;13(12):1220–2.
85. Lu X, Chittaganpitch M, Olsen SJ, et al. Real-time PCR assays for detection of bocavirus in human specimens. J Clin Microbiol 2006;44(9):3231–5.
86. Hindiyeh MY, Keller N, Mandelboim M, et al. High rate of human bocavirus and adenovirus coinfection in hospitalized Israeli children. J Clin Microbiol 2008;46(1):334–7.
87. Hamano-Hasegawa K, Morozumi M, Nakayama E, et al. Comprehensive detection of causative pathogens using real-time PCR to diagnose pediatric community-acquired pneumonia. J Infect Chemother 2008;14(6):424–32.
88. Koskenvuo M, Mottonen M, Rahiala J, et al. Respiratory viral infections in children with leukemia. Pediatr Infect Dis J 2008;27(11):974–80.
89. Regamey N, Frey U, Deffernez C, et al. Isolation of human bocavirus from Swiss infants with respiratory infections. Pediatr Infect Dis J 2007;26(2):177–9.

90. Qu XW, Duan ZJ, Qi ZY, et al. Human bocavirus infection, People's Republic of China. Emerg Infect Dis 2007;13(1):165–8.
91. Schenk T, Huck B, Forster J, et al. Human bocavirus DNA detected by quantitative real-time PCR in two children hospitalized for lower respiratory tract infection. Eur J Clin Microbiol Infect Dis 2007;26(2):147–9.
92. Regamey N, Kaiser L, Roiha HL, et al. Viral etiology of acute respiratory infections with cough in infancy: a community-based birth cohort study. Pediatr Infect Dis J 2008;27(2):100–5.
93. Esposito S, Bosis S, Niesters HG, et al. Impact of human bocavirus on children and their families. J Clin Microbiol 2008;46(4):1337–42.
94. Ziegler S, Tillmann RL, Muller A, et al. No gastroenteric Bocavirus in high risk patients stool samples. J Clin Virol 2008;43(3):349–50.
95. Tillmann RL, Simon A, Muller A, et al. Sensitive commercial NASBA assay for the detection of respiratory syncytial virus in clinical specimen. PLoS ONE 2007; 2(12):e1357.
96. Moore C, Corden S, Sinha J, et al. Dry cotton or flocked respiratory swabs as a simple collection technique for the molecular detection of respiratory viruses using real-time NASBA. J Virol Methods 2008;153(2):84–9.
97. Williams JM. 2009 update in prevention, evaluation, and outpatient treatment of influenza. Curr Med Res Opin 2009;25(4):817–28.
98. Rodriguez WJ, Gruber WC, Welliver RC, et al. Respiratory syncytial virus (RSV) immune globulin intravenous therapy for RSV lower respiratory tract infection in infants and young children at high risk for severe RSV infections: Respiratory Syncytial Virus Immune Globulin Study Group. Pediatrics 1997;99(3):454–61.
99. Orange JS, Hossny EM, Weiler CR, et al. Use of intravenous immunoglobulin in human disease: a review of evidence by members of the Primary Immunodeficiency Committee of the American Academy of Allergy, Asthma and Immunology. J Allergy Clin Immunol 2006;117(Suppl 4):S525–53.
100. Kupfer B, Vehreschild J, Cornely O, et al. Severe pneumonia and human bocavirus in adult. Emerg Infect Dis 2006;12(10):1614–6.
101. Calvo C, Garcia-Garcia ML, Blanco C, et al. Human bocavirus infection in a neonatal intensive care unit. J Infect 2008;57(3):269–71.
102. Arnold JC, Singh KK, Spector SA, et al. Undiagnosed respiratory viruses in children. Pediatrics 2008;121(3):e631–7.
103. Fabbiani M, Terrosi C, Martorelli B, et al. Epidemiological and clinical study of viral respiratory tract infections in children from Italy. J Med Virol 2009;81(4): 750–6.
104. Lin JH, Chiu SC, Lin YC, et al. Clinical and genetic analysis of Human Bocavirus in children with lower respiratory tract infection in Taiwan. J Clin Virol 2009;44(3): 219–24.
105. Norja P, Ubillos I, Templeton K, et al. No evidence for an association between infections with WU and KI polyomaviruses and respiratory disease. J Clin Virol 2007;40(4):307–11.
106. Villa L, Melon S, Suarez S, et al. Detection of human bocavirus in Asturias, Northern Spain. Eur J Clin Microbiol Infect Dis 2008;27(3):237–9.
107. Smuts H, Hardie D. Human bocavirus in hospitalized children, South Africa. Emerg Infect Dis 2006;12(9):1457–8.
108. Smuts H, Workman L, Zar HJ. Role of human metapneumovirus, human coronavirus NL63 and human bocavirus in infants and young children with acute wheezing. J Med Virol 2008;80(5):906–12.

Recently Discovered Human Coronaviruses

Brigitte A. Wevers, MSc[a], Lia van der Hoek, PhD[b,*]

KEYWORDS

- Coronaviruses • Human coronavirus 229E
- Human coronavirus NL63 • Human coronavirus OC43
- Human coronavirus HKU1
- Severe acute respiratory syndrome-associated coronavirus

Coronaviruses (CoVs) are a large and diverse group of positive-stranded RNA viruses in the *Coronaviridae* family, which also comprises members of the *Torovirus* genera.[1] Together with the *Arteriviridae* and *Roniviridae* families, *Coronaviridae* are grouped in the order of *Nidovirales*, based on their conserved genome organization and mechanism of replication.[2] The name Nidovirus is derived from their unique transcription strategy involving formation of nested (in Latin: nidus) mRNA molecules with identical 3′ ends during an infection.[3,4] Coronavirus particles are enveloped and measure 120 to 160 nm in diameter, containing a linear, single and positive stranded RNA genome with an average length of 27 to 31 kb, the largest RNA genome described so far.[2,5] The viral RNA molecule is organized together with multiple copies of the nucleocapsid (N) protein to form a flexible core inside the viral membrane that constitutes the spike (S), envelope (E), and membrane (M) proteins. In certain isolates, an additional structural protein is present on the virion: hemagglutinin esterase (HE). The heavily glycosylated S proteins are crucial for CoVs to establish and maintain an infection cycle, by interacting with specific cellular entry molecules to initiate a fusion between viral and cellular membranes.[6]

In the 1930s, isolation of the first CoV, avian bronchitis virus (IBV), was reported.[7] Ever since, many CoVs have been discovered in a broad range of hosts, including mammals and birds. CoVs are transmitted by means of respiratory aerosols and the fecal–oral route of infection, and primarily target mucosal surfaces of respiratory and intestinal tracts, causing illnesses of varying severity. In addition, manifestations

Lia van der Hoek is supported by VIDI grant 016.066.318 from the Netherlands Organization for Scientific Research (NWO).

[a] Master Biomedical Sciences, Department of Medical Microbiology, VU University Amsterdam, Faculty of Earth and Life Sciences, Amsterdam, The Netherlands
[b] Laboratory of Experimental Virology, Department of Medical Microbiology, Center for Infection and Immunity (CINIMA), Academic Medical Center (AMC), Meibergdreef 15, 1105AZ, Amsterdam, The Netherlands
* Corresponding author.
E-mail address: c.m.vanderhoek@amc.uva.nl (L. van der Hoek).

Clin Lab Med 29 (2009) 715–724
doi:10.1016/j.cll.2009.07.007
0272-2712/09/$ – see front matter © 2009 Elsevier Inc. All rights reserved.

labmed.theclinics.com

of neurologic, hepatic, and systemic disorders are induced after infection with certain CoVs.[8]

Human CoV (HCoV) infections initially seemed to be associated primarily with mild and self-limiting upper respiratory tract infections, such as the common cold, and were not thought to be connected to severe human illnesses.[9] Coronaviral pathogens however, gained renewed scientific interest in 2003, when a novel HCoV was proven to be the etiologic agent of the worldwide severe acute respiratory syndrome (SARS) epidemic.[10–14] Infection with SARS-CoV resulted in severe lower respiratory tract infections, causing high morbidity and mortality within a short period of time.[15] Soon thereafter, numerous new CoVs were discovered, including two species with the potential to infect humans: HCoV-NL63 and HCoV-HKU1.[16–18]

HUMAN CORONAVIRUS 229E AND HUMAN CORONAVIRUS OC43: COMMON COLD AGENTS

For a long time, only two HCoV species were known: HCoV-229E and HCoV-OC43, both isolated in the mid-1960s. HCoV-229E was recovered from medical students in Chicago who had clinical symptoms of upper respiratory tract infection. The virus could be propagated on primary human kidney cells and human embryonic lung cells.[19] Shortly thereafter, a distinct CoV was isolated using human embryonic tracheal organ cultures, and termed OC43 for organ culture number 43.[20] Inoculation of volunteers at the Common Cold Unit in Salisbury, United Kingdom, demonstrated a causal relationship between HCoV-229E and HCoV-OC43 infections and common cold symptoms.[21]

The common cold is a typical self-limiting upper respiratory tract disease, character-ized by mild clinical symptoms, including nasal obstruction and rhinorrhea, sneezing, sore throat, and cough. There is no single cause for this heterogeneous group of upper respiratory tract illnesses; in fact numerous viruses from several different families func-tion as etiologic agents.[22] Although rhinoviruses account for the largest proportion of all upper respiratory tract infections, HCoV-229E and HCoV-OC43 now are known to be responsible for a high number of these cases, which occur mainly during winter and early spring seasons in temperate climate countries.[23–25] Although coryza occurs more often during HCoV-229E infections, there are indications that sore throat manifes-tations are observed more frequently in patients who have HCoV-OC43 infections.[26] Infants, elderly, and immunocompromised individuals are thought to be vulnerable for more severe upper and lower respiratory tract infections, including pneumonia, caused by infections with HCoV-229E and HCoV-OC43.[9,27,28]

Since their discovery, other pathologies have been connected occasionally to HCoV-OC43 and HCoV-229E. HCoV-OC43 initially was proposed to be involved in gastrointestinal (GI) disease development in children.[29] This hypothesis, however, never was confirmed by inoculation studies with healthy individuals.[9] In addition, presence of CoV RNA in brain tissue and antibody concentrations in serum of multiple sclerosis (MS) patients, led to the suggestion of CoV involvement in MS etiology.[30–33] Although evidence for a significant correlation between presence of HCoV-229E and HCoV-OC43 RNA and MS has not been demonstrated,[34,35] accumulating recent data from cell culture and animal models indeed confirm their neurotropic and neuroinva-sive potential.[36,37] Nevertheless, actual brain invasion in MS patients by HCoV-229E and HCoV-OC43 might be explained by a disrupted blood–brain barrier.[9]

SEVERE ACUTE RESPIRATORY SYNDROME

The first case of SARS, a severe lower respiratory tract illness with a mortality rate of 10%, emerged in November 2002 in Fushan City, China.[38] Subsequently, SARS spread rapidly throughout eastern Asia and to 28 other regions around the world, causing 774 deaths in 8098 infected individuals.[39] In February 2003, a newly emerged HCoV, which originated from a wild animal reservoir, was demonstrated to be the etiologic agent of this syndrome.[11] Of all HCoVs described thus far, SARS-CoV causes the most severe clinical symptoms. Of interest, SARS rarely is detected in young children, and if so, it seems to follow a less aggressive clinical course.[40] The strongest predictor of poor disease outcome appears to be an advanced age (older than 60 years).[41]

By means of droplet inhalation, SARS-CoV reaches the respiratory tract and invades epithelial cells of trachea, bronchi, bronchioles, and alveoli.[42] SARS-CoV typically causes a broad spectrum of disease, starting with an influenza-like syndrome, including symptoms such as high fever, malaise, rigors, and fatigue.[41] After disease onset, infections may progress to a nonsevere variant of disease or cough variant, characterized by relatively moderate symptoms.[43] Generally, 2 to 7 days after SARS onset, a typical respiratory phase is initiated, including nonproductive cough and dyspnea. In two thirds of infected patients, disease deteriorates toward an atypical pneumonia, with shortness of breath and poor alveolar oxygen exchange.[44] Symptoms may worsen even further into an acute respiratory distress syndrome (ARDS), as a result of progressive pulmonary immune infiltration, formation of hyaline membranes, diffuse alveolar damage (DAD), and a high viral burden.[42,45,46] ARDS is the most severe form of acute lung injury (ALI) and is regarded as the leading cause of death in SARS-CoV infected individuals.[47,48] Lung injury in patients who have SARS is supposed to occur directly, by viral-mediated destruction of alveolar and bronchial epithelial cells, as well as indirectly, through extensive production of immune mediators.[41,44]

HUMAN CORONAVIRUS NL63 AND HUMAN CORONAVIRUS HKU1 INFECTIONS

Shortly after the SARS-CoV outbreak, an unknown respiratory virus was isolated in Amsterdam, The Netherlands, in a nasopharyngeal aspirate specimen (sample NL63) from a 7-month-old infant suffering from coryza, bronchiolitis, conjunctivitis, and fever. The infectious agent was identified as a distinct and fourth human member of the *Coronaviridae* family: HCoV-NL63, using a novel technique to amplify viral genomes without a priori knowledge of their sequence.[17] Within a few weeks, a second research group from The Netherlands reported detection of essentially the same virus, initially designated HCoV-NL.[16] Because similarity of these isolates is very high at the nucleotide level, they both represent the same species: HCoV-NL63. HCoV-NL63 is demonstrated to be genetically most closely related to HCoV-229E.[49] HCoV-NL63 infections are recognized throughout the whole world, and are identified as nonfatal upper and lower respiratory tract infections in infants, the elderly, and immunocompromised adults.[9] In addition, a clear association between HCoV-NL63 infections and trachea inflammation in children (laryngotracheitis or croup) has been demonstrated through population-based studies.[50–53] In patients who have croup, HCoV-NL63 infections are detected as frequently as the parainfluenzaviruses, which initially were considered as the main causative agent for this illness.[50] Although an additional fascinating disease association was proposed for HCoV-NL63 and Kawasaki disease (the most common form of childhood vasculitis),[54] it could not be confirmed by subsequent investigations.[55–60] Several current indications strongly suggest that HCoV-NL63, in addition to HCoV-229E and HCoV-OC43, is a common cold-causing virus in healthy adults. Actual evidence for this causal relationship is, unfortunately, still lacking.

In January 2005, a fifth HCoV was discovered in Hong Kong, China. HCoV-HKU1 was recovered from an adult who had chronic pulmonary disease, and it was only distantly related to HCoV-OC43.[18] Clinical symptoms accompanying an HCoV-HKU1 infection include rhinorrhea, fever, cough, febrile seizure, wheezing, pneumonia, and bronchiolitis.[18,61] Similar to HCoV-NL63, infections with HCoV-HKU1 have been detected worldwide; they presumably are associated with common colds, and most likely cause a more severe clinical spectrum of respiratory disease in young children, adults with underlying disease, or the elderly.[62] Furthermore, there are indications that HCoV-HKU1 also might play a role in GI disease.[63]

KOCH'S POSTULATES

Once novel viruses are identified, it is important to demonstrate their pathogenic potential and unravel a causal link with a specific disease. Proof of such a relationship ideally would imply fulfilling Koch's postulates, which have been revisited for viral pathogens.[64] These standard criteria propose that a causal connection between a new virus and an illness may be established if:

The organism is consistently present in patients who have disease at a higher prevalence than in control patients.
The disease is replicated in an appropriate animal model after viral challenge, and subsequently isolated from this animal.
A specific host immune response can be demonstrated.

In the case of HCoV-NL63 and HCoV-HKU1, application of all Koch's postulates turned out to be impossible, and their role in disease therefore remains unconfirmed. Currently, HCoV-HKU1 cannot be maintained in cell culture systems, and animal models are unavailable for both NL63 and HKU1 CoVs. Animal model systems susceptible for HCoV-OC43 and SARS-CoV have been developed previously, and allow present studies of coronaviral tropism, replication, recombination, and accompanying immune modulatory mechanisms.[65,66] Most recently, a very important technical achievement has been made for studying pathogenic mechanisms of HCoV-NL63, because infectious full-length cDNA clones of the HCoV-NL63 genome can be engineered.[67] Nonetheless, thus far, the only option to identify pathogenic potential of HCoV-NL63 and HCoV-HKU1 is to determine a significant association with a disease through epidemiologic studies with proper control groups.[9] An alternative strategy to gain novel insights in mechanisms of CoV pathogenesis is by extensive characterization of virus–host interactions and host cell invasion strategies. Viral receptor specificity and expression are generally important determinants of the pathogenic potential of a virus and the nature of the disease that it causes.[68]

CELLULAR RECEPTOR MODULATION: A PATHWAY TO HUMAN CORONAVIRUS PATHOGENESIS

Viral receptors, components that actively promote host cell entry, differ greatly from one virus to the next and constitute a wide variety of proteins and carbohydrates, each with distinct physiologic functions.[68] Although cellular receptors for HCoV-OC43 and HCoV-HKU1 remain to be elucidated, the family of membrane-associated proteases seems to be favored by HCoVs, because both neutral aminopeptidase (APN), the receptor for HCoV-229E,[69] and angiotensin-converting enzyme 2 (ACE2), the receptor for SARS-CoV and HCoV-NL63,[70–72] exist as prominent zinc-dependent peptidases on host cell plasma membranes.[73,74] In fact, several structural features of zinc metallopeptidases probably facilitate targeting of APN and ACE2 and govern ellular entry of HCoVs. Zinc peptidases are expressed abundantly on various cell types, because these proteases modulate activity of many proteins including membrane proteins and circulating regulatory peptides.[75] Furthermore, both APN and ACE2 appear as heavy glycosylated ectoenzymes, with most of the protein, including catalytic domain, protruding into the extracellular space.[73]

During establishment of an infection, interaction of HCoV-229E and SARS-CoV spike proteins with APN or ACE2, respectively, causes a substantial modulation of these cellular entry receptors.[76–78] SARS-CoV has been proven to induce a rapid down-regulation of ACE2 cell surface expression, preferably by means of internalization of the receptor–ligand complex.[78,79] Alternatively, SARS-CoV possesses the capacity to abrogate ACE2 cell surface expression by means of activation of tumor necrosis factor-alpha converting enzyme (TACE). This enzyme mediates ectodomain shedding of ACE2.[80,81] Whether HCoV-NL63 induces a similar down-regulation of ACE2 during infection is at present unknown.

It is assumed that cellular APN expression is altered during establishment of an HCoV-229E infection. Following HCoV-229E binding to the target cell, APN molecules aggregate and translocate to caveolin-enriched membrane domains, to activate a specialized endocytic route of virus particle internalization.[77] Most importantly, these processes of receptor-mediated endocytosis often involve simultaneous internalization of the cellular entry molecule itself.[82,83] Likewise, sequestration of porcine APN molecules into intracellular vesicles has been visualized during endocytosis of CoV strain porcine-transmissible gastroenteritis virus (TGEV).[84] Thus, HCoV-229E-induced abrogation of APN expression is highly plausible to occur, although direct evidence is unavailable. Viral targeting of APN and its subsequent down-regulation is definitely a known phenomenon, as this cellular peptidase possibly is implicated in infection with human cytomegalovirus (CMV) also.[85–87] Notwithstanding the fact that human APN is most likely not the primary receptor of the virus,[88] CMV induces abrogation of APN expression.[85,86]

The phenomenon of entry receptor suppression has been reported for several additional viruses, including HIV, measles virus (MV), influenza virus, and human herpes virus (HHV) type 6.[89–92] Although it may seem contradictory, viruses strongly benefit from down-regulation of their own receptors, and this process correlates with an enhanced pathogenesis also.[93] Abrogation of receptor expression prevents infection of cells by additional virus particles in which viral replication is already progressing.[94] In addition to limiting superinfection, receptor down-regulation can facilitate efficient virion release, leading to a controlled and productive infection.[95] At the same time, abrogation of receptor expression hampers natural physiologic activity of these cellular molecules and therefore may contribute to viral disease pathogenesis also. Internalization of CD4 after HIV-gp120 binding, for example, leads to specific impairment of immune cell functions.[96] Moreover, MV hemagglutinin (HA)-induced CD46 receptor abrogation induces serious dysregulation of complement pathways and mechanisms of immunosuppression.[97,98]

Down-regulation of APN and ACE2 during HCoV-229E, HCoV-NL63, and SARS-CoV infection may impair the normal physiologic function of the host cells severely and contribute to the development of clinical manifestations. Besides their classification as zinc-dependent peptidases, APN and ACE2 share important functional enzymatic characteristics. Both proteins are integral components of the renin–angiotensin system (RAS). This endocrine system is one of the most important regulators of human physiology, with a key role in maintenance of arterial pressure, fluid hemostatis, salt balances, cardiac function, cell proliferation and hypertrophy, angiogenesis, and apoptosis. Therefore, impaired expression of APN and ACE2 also might alter crucial normal physiologic functionalities of the RAS. Most intriguingly, suppression of ACE₂ protein expression during SARS-CoV infection actually causes severe imbalances within the enzymatic RAS cascade, which is proposed to be the main cause of severe acute pneumonia and acute lung failure observed during SARS-CoV infection.[71,76,99] These findings raise the possibility that CoV-induced dysregulation of the RAS might be important for the clinical outcome of HCoV-229E and HCoV-NL63 infections also.

SUMMARY

CoVs are recognized human pathogens, associated with relatively mild upper respiratory tract infections in healthy adults and more serious respiratory complications in weakened patients. A virus-induced modulation of receptor expression could be involved in the onset of CoV-associated clinical symptoms, and future research should focus on elucidation of the physiologic consequences following virus–host interactions. Insight into these processes would contribute to the clarification of the strategies used by HCoVs to elicit specific diseases and might provide a definite demonstration of their etiology also. Eventually, a better understanding of HCoV pathogenesis may lead to development of new therapeutic strategies.

REFERENCES

1. Gonzalez JM, Gomez-Puertas P, Cavanagh D, et al. A comparative sequence analysis to revise the current taxonomy of the family Coronaviridae. Arch Virol 2003;148(11):2207–35.
2. Gorbalenya AE, Enjuanes L, Ziebuhr J, et al. Nidovirales: evolving the largest RNA virus genome. Virus Res 2006;117(1):17–37.
3. Pasternak AO, Spaan WJ, Snijder EJ. Nidovirus transcription: how to make sense...? J Gen Virol 2006;87:1403–21.
4. Sawicki SG, Sawicki DL, Siddell SG. A contemporary view of coronavirus transcription. J Virol 2007;81(1):20–9.
5. Masters PS. The molecular biology of coronaviruses. Adv Virus Res 2006;66: 193–292.
6. Gallagher TM, Buchmeier MJ. Coronavirus spike proteins in viral entry and pathogenesis. Virology 2001;279(2):371–4.
7. Lai MMC, Perlman S, Anderson LJ. Coronaviridae. In: Knipe MD, Howley PM, editors. Field's virology. Philadelphia: Lippincott Williams & Wilkins; 2007. p. 1305–56.
8. McIntosh K. Coronaviruses. In: Knipe DM, Howley PM, editors. Field's virology. Philadelphia: Lippincott-Raven Publishers; 1996. p. 1095–103.
9. van der Hoek L. Human coronaviruses: what do they cause? Antivir Ther 2007; 12(4 Pt B):651–8.
10. Drosten C, Gunther S, Preiser W, et al. Identification of a novel coronavirus in patients with severe acute respiratory syndrome. N Engl J Med 2003;348(20): 1967–76.
11. Fouchier RA, Kuiken T, Schutten M, et al. Aetiology: Koch's postulates fulfilled for SARS virus [letter]. Nature 2003;423(6937):240.
12. Ksiazek TG, Erdman D, Goldsmith CS, et al. A novel coronavirus associated with severe acute respiratory syndrome. N Engl J Med 2003;348(20):1953–66.
13. Kuiken T, Fouchier RA, Schutten M, et al. Newly discovered coronavirus as the primary cause of severe acute respiratory syndrome. Lancet 2003;362(9380): 263–70.
14. Peiris JS, Lai ST, Poon LL, et al. Coronavirus as a possible cause of severe acute respiratory syndrome. Lancet 2003;361(9366):1319–25.

15. Peiris JS, Guan Y, Yuen KY. Severe acute respiratory syndrome. Nat Med 2004; 10(Suppl 12):s88–97.
16. Fouchier RA, Hartwig NG, Bestebroer TM, et al. A previously undescribed coronavirus associated with respiratory disease in humans. Proc Natl Acad Sci U S A 2004;101(16):6212–6.
17. van der Hoek L, Pyrc K, Jebbink MF, et al. Identification of a new human coronavirus. Nat Med 2004;10(4):368–73.
18. Woo PC, Lau SK, Chu CM, et al. Characterization and complete genome sequence of a novel coronavirus, coronavirus HKU1, from patients with pneumonia. J Virol 2005;79(2):884–95.
19. Hamre D, Procknow JJ. A new virus isolated from the human respiratory tract. Proc Soc Exp Biol Med 1966;121(1):190–3.
20. McIntosh K, Dees JH, Becker WB, et al. Recovery in tracheal organ cultures of novel viruses from patients with respiratory disease. Proc Natl Acad Sci U S A 1967;57(4):933–40.
21. Bradburne AF, Bynoe ML, Tyrrell DA. Effects of a new human respiratory virus in volunteers. Br Med J 1967;3(5568):767–9.
22. Heikkinen T, Jarvinen A. The common cold. Lancet 2003;361(9351):51–9.
23. Larson HE, Reed SE, Tyrrell DA. Isolation of rhinoviruses and coronaviruses from 38 colds in adults. J Med Virol 1980;5(3):221–9.
24. Myint S, Johnston S, Sanderson G, et al. Evaluation of nested polymerase chain methods for the detection of human coronaviruses 229E and OC43. Mol Cell Probes 1994;8(5):357–64.
25. Navas-Martin SR, Weiss S. Coronavirus replication and pathogenesis: implications for the recent outbreak of severe acute respiratory syndrome (SARS) and the challenge for vaccine development. J Neurovirol 2004;10(2):75–85.
26. Reed SE. The behaviour of recent isolates of human respiratory coronavirus in vitro and in volunteers: evidence of heterogeneity among 229E-related strains. J Med Virol 1984;13(2):179–92.
27. Riski H, Hovi T. Coronavirus infections of man associated with diseases other than the common cold. J Med Virol 1980;6(3):259–65.
28. Kahn JS. The widening scope of coronaviruses. Curr Opin Pediatr 2006;18(1):42–7.
29. Resta S, Luby JP, Rosenfeld CR, et al. Isolation and propagation of a human enteric coronavirus. Science 1985;229(4717):978–81.
30. Burks JS, DeVald BL, Jankovsky LD, et al. Two coronaviruses isolated from central nervous system tissue of two multiple sclerosis patients. Science 1980;209(4459):933–4.
31. Murray RS, Brown B, Brian D, et al. Detection of coronavirus RNA and antigen in multiple sclerosis brain. Ann Neurol 1992;31(5):525–33.
32. Stewart JN, Mounir S, Talbot PJ. Human coronavirus gene expression in the brains of multiple sclerosis patients. Virology 1992;191(1):502–5.
33. Arbour N, Day R, Newcombe J, et al. Neuroinvasion by human respiratory coronaviruses. J Virol 2000;74(19):8913–21.
34. Dessau RB, Lisby G, Frederiksen JL. Coronaviruses in brain tissue from patients with multiple sclerosis. Acta Neuropathol 2001;101(6):601–4.
35. Gilden DH. Infectious causes of multiple sclerosis. Lancet Neurol 2005;4(3):195–202.
36. Bonavia A, Arbour N, Yong VW, et al. Infection of primary cultures of human neural cells by human coronaviruses 229E and OC43. J Virol 1997;71(1):800–6.

37. Jacomy H, Fragoso G, Almazan G, et al. Human coronavirus OC43 infection induces chronic encephalitis leading to disabilities in BALB/C mice. Virology 2006;349(2):335–46.
38. Zhao Z, Zhang F, Xu M, et al. Description and clinical treatment of an early outbreak of severe acute respiratory syndrome (SARS) in Guangzhou, PR China. J Med Microbiol 2003;52:715–20.
39. Summary of probable SARS cases with onset of illness from November 1, 2002 to July 31, 2003. Available at: http://www.who.int. Accessed February 9, 2009.
40. Hon KL, Leung CW, Cheng WT, et al. Clinical presentations and outcome of severe acute respiratory syndrome in children. Lancet 2003;361(9370):1701–3.
41. Cameron MJ, Bermejo-Martin JF, Danesh A, et al. Human immunopathogenesis of severe acute respiratory syndrome (SARS). Virus Res 2008;133(1):13–9.
42. Guo Y, Korteweg C, McNutt MA, et al. Pathogenetic mechanisms of severe acute respiratory syndrome. Virus Res 2008;133(1):4–12.
43. Christian MD, Poutanen SM, Loutfy MR, et al. Severe acute respiratory syndrome. Clin Infect Dis 2004;38(10):1420–7.
44. Perlman S, Dandekar AA. Immunopathogenesis of coronavirus infections: implications for SARS. Nat Rev Immunol 2005;5(12):917–27.
45. Fowler RA, Lapinsky SE, Hallett D, et al. Critically ill patients with severe acute respiratory syndrome. JAMA 2003;290(3):367–73.
46. Lew TW, Kwek TK, Tai D, et al. Acute respiratory distress syndrome in critically ill patients with severe acute respiratory syndrome. JAMA 2003;290(3):374–80.
47. Ware LB, Matthay MA. The acute respiratory distress syndrome. N Engl J Med 2000;342(18):1334–49.
48. Imai Y, Kuba K, Neely GG, et al. Identification of oxidative stress and toll-like receptor 4 signaling as a key pathway of acute lung injury. Cell 2008;133(2): 235–49.
49. Pyrc K, Dijkman R, Deng L, et al. Mosaic structure of human coronavirus NL63, one thousand years of evolution. J Mol Biol 2006;364(5):964–73.
50. van der Hoek L, Sure K, Ihorst G, et al. Croup is associated with the novel coronavirus NL63. PLoS Med 2005;2(8):764–70.
51. Choi EH, Lee HJ, Kim SJ, et al. The association of newly identified respiratory viruses with lower respiratory tract infections in Korean children, 2000–2005. Clin Infect Dis 2006;43(5):585–92.
52. Han TH, Chung JY, Kim SW, et al. Human coronavirus-NL63 infections in Korean children, 2004–2006. J Clin Virol 2007;38(1):27–31.
53. Wu PS, Chang LY, Berkhout B, et al. Clinical manifestations of human coronavirus NL63 infection in children in Taiwan. Eur J Pediatr 2008;167(1):75–80.
54. Esper F, Shapiro ED, Weibel C, et al. Association between a novel human coronavirus and Kawasaki disease. J Infect Dis 2005;191(4):499–502.
55. Shimizu C, Shike H, Baker SC, et al. Human coronavirus NL63 is not detected in the respiratory tracts of children with acute Kawasaki disease. J Infect Dis 2005; 192(10):1767–71.
56. Ebihara T, Endo R, Ma X, et al. Lack of association between New Haven coronavirus and Kawasaki disease. J Infect Dis 2005;192(2):351–2 [author reply 353].
57. Belay ED, Erdman DD, Anderson LJ, et al. Kawasaki disease and human coronavirus. J Infect Dis 2005;192(2):352–3 [author reply 353].
58. Chang LY, Chiang BL, Kao CL, et al. Lack of association between infection with a novel human coronavirus (HCoV), HCoV-NH, and Kawasaki disease in Taiwan. J Infect Dis 2006;193(2):283–6.

9. Dominguez SR, Anderson MS, Glode MP, et al. Blinded case–control study of the relationship between human coronavirus NL63 and Kawasaki syndrome. J Infect Dis 2006;194(12):1697–701.

0. Lehmann C, Klar R, Lindner J, et al. Kawasaki disease lacks association with human coronavirus NL63 and human bocavirus. Pediatr Infect Dis J 2009; 28(6):553–4.

1. Woo PC, Lau SK, Tsoi HW, et al. Clinical and molecular epidemiological features of coronavirus HKU1-associated community-acquired pneumonia. J Infect Dis 2005;192(11):1898–907.

2. Pyrc K, Berkhout B, van der Hoek L. The novel human coronaviruses NL63 and HKU1. J Virol 2007;81(7):3051–7.

3. Vabret A, Dina J, Gouarin S, et al. Detection of the new human coronavirus HKU1: a report of 6 cases. Clin Infect Dis 2006;42(5):634–9.

4. Fredericks DN, Relman DA. Sequence-based identification of microbial pathogens: a reconsideration of Koch's postulates. Clin Microbiol Rev 1996;9(1):18–33.

5. Jacomy H, Talbot PJ. Vacuolating encephalitis in mice infected by human coronavirus OC43. Virology 2003;315(1):20–33.

6. Roberts A, Deming D, Paddock CD, et al. A mouse-adapted SARS coronavirus causes disease and mortality in BALB/c mice. PLoS Pathog 2007;3(1):23–37.

7. Donaldson EF, Yount B, Sims AC, et al. Systematic assembly of a full-length infectious clone of human coronavirus NL63. J Virol Dec 2008;82(23):11948–57.

8. Helenius A. Virus entry and uncoating. In: Knipe MD, Howley PM, editors. Field's virology. Philadelphia: Lippincott Williams & Wilkins; 2007. p. 99–118.

9. Yeager CL, Ashmun RA, Williams RK, et al. Human aminopeptidase N is a receptor for human coronavirus 229E. Nature 1992;357(6377):420–2.

70. Li W, Moore MJ, Vasilieva N, et al. Angiotensin-converting enzyme 2 is a functional receptor for the SARS coronavirus. Nature 2003;426(6965):450–4.

71. Kuba K, Imai Y, Rao S, et al. A crucial role of angiotensin converting enzyme 2 (ACE2) in SARS coronavirus-induced lung injury. Nat Med 2005;11(8):875–9.

72. Hofmann H, Pyrc K, van der Hoek L, et al. Human coronavirus NL63 employs the severe acute respiratory syndrome coronavirus receptor for cellular entry. Proc Natl Acad Sci U S A 2005;102(22):7988–93.

73. Turner AJ, Hiscox JA, Hooper NM. ACE2: from vasopeptidase to SARS virus receptor. Trends Pharmacol Sci 2004;25(6):291–4.

74. Mina-Osorio P. The moonlighting enzyme CD13: old and new functions to target. Trends Mol Med 2008;14(8):361–71.

75. Guy JL, Lambert DW, Warner FJ, et al. Membrane-associated zinc peptidase families: comparing ACE and ACE2. Biochim Biophys Acta 2005;1751(1):2–8.

76. Imai Y, Kuba K, Penninger JM. The discovery of angiotensin-converting enzyme 2 and its role in acute lung injury in mice. Exp Physiol 2008;93(5):543–8.

77. Nomura R, Kiyota A, Suzaki E, et al. Human coronavirus 229E binds to CD13 in rafts and enters the cell through caveolae. J Virol 2004;78(16):8701–8.

78. Wang H, Yang P, Liu K, et al. SARS coronavirus entry into host cells through a novel clathrin- and caveolae-independent endocytic pathway. Cell Res 2008; 18(2):290–301.

79. Wang S, Guo F, Liu K, et al. Endocytosis of the receptor-binding domain of SARS-CoV spike protein together with virus receptor ACE2. Virus Res 2008;136:8–15.

80. Haga S, Yamamoto N, Nakai-Murakami C, et al. Modulation of TNF-alpha converting enzyme by the spike protein of SARS-CoV and ACE2 induces TNF alpha production and facilitates viral entry. Proc Natl Acad Sci U S A 2008;105(22): 7809–14.

81. Jia HP, Look DC, Tan P, et al. Ectodomain shedding of angiotensin-converting enzyme 2 in human airway epithelia. Am J Physiol Lung Cell Mol Physiol 2009; 297(1):L84–96.
82. Le Roy C, Wrana JL. Clathrin- and nonclathrin-mediated endocytic regulation of cell signaling. Nat Rev Mol Cell Biol 2005;6(2):112–26.
83. Marsh M, Helenius A. Virus entry: open sesame. Cell 2006;124(4):729–40.
84. Hansen GH, Delmas B, Besnardeau L, et al. The coronavirus- transmissible gastroenteritis virus causes infection after receptor-mediated endocytosis and acid-dependent fusion with an intracellular compartment. J Virol 1998;72(1): 527–34.
85. Gredmark S, Britt WB, Xie X, et al. Human cytomegalovirus induces inhibition of macrophage differentiation by binding to human aminopeptidase N/CD13. J Immunol 2004;173(8):4897–907.
86. Phillips AJ, Tomasec P, Wang EC, et al. Human cytomegalovirus infection down-regulates expression of the cellular aminopeptidases CD10 and CD13. Virology 1998;250(2):350–8.
87. Soderberg C, Giugni TD, Zaia JA, et al. CD13 (human aminopeptidase N) mediates human cytomegalovirus infection. J Virol 1993;67(11):6576–85.
88. Isaacson MK, Feire AL, Compton T. Epidermal growth factor receptor is not required for human cytomegalovirus entry or signaling. J Virol 2007;81(12): 6241–7.
89. Aiken C, Konner J, Landau NR, et al. Nef induces CD4 endocytosis: requirement for a critical dileucine motif in the membrane-proximal CD4 cytoplasmic domain. Cell 1994;76(5):853–64.
90. Schneider-Schaulies J, Schnorr JJ, Brinckmann U, et al. Receptor usage and differential down-regulation of CD46 by measles virus wild-type and vaccine strains. Proc Natl Acad Sci U S A 1995;92(9):3943–7.
91. Marschall M, Meier-Ewert H, Herrler G, et al. The cell receptor level is reduced during persistent infection with influenza C virus. Arch Virol 1997;142(6):1155–64.
92. Santoro F, Kennedy PE, Locatelli G, et al. CD46 is a cellular receptor for human herpesvirus 6. Cell 1999;99(7):817–27.
93. Stoddart CA, Geleziunas R, Ferrell S, et al. Human immunodeficiency virus type 1 Nef-mediated down-regulation of CD4 correlates with Nef enhancement of viral pathogenesis. J Virol 2003;77(3):2124–33.
94. Michel N, Allespach I, Venzke S, et al. The Nef protein of human immunodeficiency virus establishes superinfection immunity by a dual strategy to down-regulate cell surface CCR5 and CD4. Curr Biol 2005;15(8):714–23.
95. Ross TM, Oran AE, Cullen BR. Inhibition of HIV-1 progeny virion release by cell-surface CD4 is relieved by expression of the viral Nef protein. Curr Biol 1999; 9(12):613–21.
96. Wahl SM, Allen JB, Gartner S, et al. HIV-1 and its envelope glycoprotein down-regulate chemotactic ligand receptors and chemotactic function of peripheral blood monocytes. J Immunol 1989;142(10):3553–9.
97. Oldstone MB, Lewicki H, Thomas D, et al. Measles virus infection in a transgenic model: virus-induced immunosuppression and central nervous system disease. Cell 1999;98(5):629–40.
98. Schnorr JJ, Dunster LM, Nanan R, et al. Measles virus-induced down-regulation of CD46 is associated with enhanced sensitivity to complement-mediated lysis of infected cells. Eur J Immunol 1995;25(4):976–84.
99. Imai Y, Kuba K, Rao S, et al. Angiotensin-converting enzyme 2 protects from severe acute lung failure. Nature 2005;436(7047):112–6.

Respiratory Syncytial Virus Vaccine Development

Yoshihiko Murata, MD, PhD[a,b,*]

KEYWORDS

- Respiratory syncytial virus • Vaccine • Humoral immunity
- Cellular immunity • Respiratory tract infection

Since its identification in 1956, respiratory syncytial virus (RSV) has been known to be a significant cause of respiratory tract illness in persons of all ages, and it is the most clinically important cause of lower respiratory tract infections in infants and children.[1] Following primary RSV infection, which generally occurs by age 2, immunity to RSV remains incomplete, and frequent reinfections occur throughout life, with the most severe infections occurring at the extremes of age and among the immunocompromised.[2] In the United States, RSV is estimated to cause approximately 126,000 annual hospitalizations and approximately 300 deaths among infants younger than 1 year old.[3] Furthermore, RSV accounts for more than 80,000 hospitalizations and more than13,000 deaths each winter among adults who are elderly or have underlying cardiopulmonary or immunosuppressive conditions.[4] Despite such burden of disease, the number of currently licensed prophylactic and therapeutic agents against RSV infection remains exceedingly limited—the humanized monoclonal antibody (mAb) palivizumab, which is licensed only for use in high-risk infants, and ribavirin, which is licensed for use only in the pediatric population.[1] Because of marked imbalance between the clinical burden of RSV and the available therapeutic and prophylactic options, development of an RSV vaccine remains an unmet medical need (**Table 1**).

RSV is an enveloped virus of the *Paramyxoviridae* family.[5] Clinical RSV isolates are classified according to antigenic group (A or B) and further subdivided into five to six genotypes based on the genetic variability within the viral genome. Each virion contains a nonsegmented, negative sense, single-stranded RNA that encodes 11 proteins, eight being structural and three nonstructural (NS1, NS2, M2-2). The viral

This work was supported by Grant Number AI076781 from the National Institutes of Health. Dr. Murata is also a coauthor of a provisional patent application on the use of human papillomavirus L1 capsid protein and its derivatives as respiratory syncytial virus vaccine candidates.

[a] Division of Infectious Diseases, Department of Medicine, University of Rochester School of Medicine and Dentistry, 575 Elmwood Avenue, Box 689, Rochester, NY 14642, USA
[b] Infectious Diseases Unit, Rochester General Hospital, 1425 Portland Avenue, Rochester, NY 14621, USA
* Division of Infectious Diseases, Department of Medicine, University of Rochester School of Medicine and Dentistry, 575 Elmwood Avenue, Box 689, Rochester, NY 14642.
E-mail address: Yoshihiko_Murata@urmc.rochester.edu

Table 1
Overview of various experimental approaches to respiratory syncytial virus vaccine development

Experimental Approach	Preclinical Study Comments	Clinical Study Comments
Nonreplicating, inactivated virus		
Formalin-inactivated		Associated with potentiation of respiratory syncytial virus (RSV) disease among RSV-naïve infants and children; testing discontinued
Subunit-based		
Purified RSV F protein		Elicits anti-RSV antibodies in RSV-seropositive children and adults
		In general, an inverse correlation between homogeneity of RSV F protein preparation and subsequent immunogenicity
F/G/M coformulation		Phase 2 testing: immunogenic in healthy and elderly high-risk adults
Bacterially derived RSV G derivative	Confers protection in rodent models despite modest levels of RSV-neutralizing antibodies	Phase 2 testing: immunogenic Phase 3 testing: discontinued
RSV F and G proteins purified from RSV-infected cells	In general: elicits poorly neutralizing antibodies and can lead to pulmonary pathology reminiscent of formalin-inactivated RSV in animal models	
	Use of toll-like receptor agonists may significantly alter immunogenicity and adverse effects in rodent models	
Virus-like particles	Hepatitis B surface antigen derivatives bearing RSV M2 cytotoxic T lymphocyte epitope generated	
	RSV nucleocapsid protein complexes elicit protective efficacy in mice	

		Phase 1/2 studies started but not reported
F/G chimeric proteins		
RSV F- and G-derived peptides	Short F-derived fragments fused to cholera holotoxin elicited RSV-neutralizing antibodies and modest protective efficacy in mice RSV G-derived peptides generated protective efficacy despite limited RSV neutralizing response in mice	
Vector-based		
Vaccinia virus expressing RSV F and G	No significant immunogenicity or protective efficacy in primates	
Adenovirus expressing RSV F	No significant immunogenicity or protective efficacy in primates	
Human parainfluenza virus 3, Sendai virus, bovine parainfluenza virus (BPIV)/HPIV 3 expressing RSV F and G	BPIV3 + RSV F immunogenic and efficacious in primates	Currently under clinical investigation
Staphylococcus carnosus expressing portions of RSV G	Limited and variable protective efficacy in mice	
RSV F and G expressed using replication-noncompetent alphavirus vectors, avian Newcastle disease virus, human rhinovirus 14	Immunogenic and protective to varying degrees in mice	
DNA-based		
DNA plasmids expressing RSV F or G	Various routes of administration Immunogenic and protective to varying degrees in animal models	
Live-attenuated and genetically engineered RSV derivatives		
Cold-passaged (cp) and temperature-sensitive (ts) phenotypes		Immunogenic in RSV-naïve and −seropositive subjects
Second-generation derivatives (bearing gene deletions or attenuating mutations) based on reverse genetics		Challenges of phenotype (over- or underattenuation in clinical studies) and genotype (genetic instability/variability during host replication)

envelope bears three transmembrane glycoproteins (G, F, SH) and the matrix (M) protein. Within the envelope, viral RNA is encapsidated by a transcriptase complex comprised of the N (nucleocapsid), P (phosphoprotein), M2-1 (transcription elongation factor), and L (polymerase) proteins. The early events in RSV replication are: viral attachment to the target cell, a process mediated mainly by the attachment (G) glycoprotein, and membrane fusion and viral penetration into the host cell, processes that require the fusion (F) protein and are augmented by the SH protein. Among viral isolates, some RSV-encoded proteins such as F are conserved highly with respect to amino acid (aa) sequence, while others such as G display extensive antigenic variation between and within the two major antigenic groups.

The various RSV-encoded proteins have been analyzed extensively with respect to their immunogenicity. Several proteins, including N, M2-1, NS1, and F, bear epitopes that induce cytotoxic T lymphocyte (CTL) responses in murine- or human-derived lymphocytes.[5] In contrast, extensive efforts to identify CTL epitopes in other proteins, including the G protein, have been unfruitful. With regard to humoral response, only antibodies against F or G are neutralizing and confer resistance to RSV upon passive transfer in animal models.[6,7] Several F-specific neutralizing mAbs also possess the ability to inhibit viral fusion activity.[8] One such mAb is palivizumab, a humanized derivative of an anti-F neutralizing mAb that is licensed for prevention of serious RSV illness in high-risk children.[9]

RESPIRATORY SYNCYTIAL VIRUS IMMUNE RESPONSES—BALANCE BETWEEN PROTECTION AND DISEASE PATHOGENESIS

In the infected host, RSV stimulates a broad range of innate and adaptive immune responses, including chemokine and cytokine secretion and neutralizing humoral and mucosal antibodies and type 1 and type 2 CD4+ and CD8+ T cells.[5,10] These host immune responses, in turn, are thought to be primarily responsible for the clinical manifestations of RSV infections, because RSV causes limited cell cytopathology in vivo.[10] Based on extensive testing in animal models and also from human immunologic studies, the phenotypic manifestations and severity of RSV disease are mediated by the fine balance and dynamic interactions among the various chemokine, cytokine, and cellular responses.[11]

Within the host, cellular and humoral responses appear to play different roles in the protection against and resolution of RSV infection and disease pathogenesis. As shown by clinical and preclinical studies with palivizumab, RSV-specific antibodies are sufficient to prevent or limit the severity of infection but are not required for clearing primary infection.[9] Once RSV infection is established, however, T cell-mediated responses are necessary to abolish viral replication.[12] In murine models, passive transfer of CD4+ T cells and CD8+ CTL eliminates RSV, the latter being more efficacious.[13] Additionally, T cell responses play key roles in pulmonary pathology during infection, with striking differences noted between interferon-γ (IFN-γ) secreting CD4+ T cells (Th1) and interleukin (IL)-4 secreting CD4+ cells (Th2). Th1, with or without associated CD8+ CTL response, clear virus with minimal lung pathology, while viral clearance by Th2 is associated with more significant pulmonary changes, often marked by eosinophilic infiltration.[14,15]

Of profound relevance to vaccine design is the effect of the priming immune response on clinical illness and lung pathology during subsequent RSV infection. Immunization with live RSV or with replicating vectors encoding RSV F protein induces a Th1-dominant response with neutralizing antibody and CD8+ CTL responses that are associated with minimal pulmonary pathology upon virus challenge.[11,16]

In contrast, immunization with inactivated RSV preparation induces a Th2-dominant response without associated CD8+ CTL but paradoxically leads to increased pathologic changes in the lungs.[17] Interestingly, the administration of RSV G protein as a purified subunit vaccine or even in the context of a replicating vector induces a Th2-dominant response and leads to eosinophilic pulmonary infiltrates and airway hyper-reactivity following virus challenge.[18] It should be noted that these observations are strikingly reminiscent of the first RSV vaccine studies using formalin-inactivated virus.

FACTORS TO BE CONSIDERED FOR RESPIRATORY SYNCYTIAL VIRUS VACCINE DEVELOPMENT

Extensive review of RSV replication, pathogenesis, and immune response in animal models and human infections has identified several key issues for RSV vaccine development.[19] First, the immune system of young infants, the primary population for vaccination, is notable for its immaturity and the presence of maternal anti-RSV antibodies during the first several months of life; in turn, these two factors may negatively affect the emergence of a robust immune response following vaccination. Second, a successful RSV vaccine must be able to target both A and B subtypes; this requirement is hampered by the genetic variability of RSV genome, and particularly of the RSV G protein, and the post-translational glycosylation of F and G proteins. Third, immunity against RSV remains incomplete after natural infection, and thus annual vaccinations may be required; the goal of such vaccination programs is to prevent severe lower respiratory tract infections. It is possible that two vaccines—one for the RSV-naïve, infant population and another for RSV-experienced adults—may be required. Lastly, in the historical context of formalin-inactivated RSV vaccine trials, the safety profile of RSV vaccine candidates will need to be well established during preclinical and clinical development.

PRIOR AND CURRENT RESPIRATORY SYNCYTIAL VIRUS VACCINE APPROACHES

Various strategies have been pursued to develop an effective and safe RSV vaccine including: inactivated virus preparations, live attenuated/genetically engineered viruses, purified RSV protein subunit vaccine preparations, vector-based vaccine candidates, and DNA-based vaccines. Each approach will be summarized.

Inactivated Virus Preparations

The first vaccine trial, performed nearly 40 years ago, employed a formalin-inactivated whole virus preparation (FI-RSV) with aluminum hydroxide adjuvant.[20] Strikingly, FI-RSV failed to induce neutralizing antibodies or protect vaccinated infants and unexpectedly led to enhanced disease severity when RSV infection occurred during the subsequent winter; in one center, more than 80% of the recipients of the FI-RSV vaccine required hospitalization as compared with only 5% of RSV-infected control subjects.[21–23] Such disease enhancement, or potentiation, in which the vaccination paradoxically worsened the clinical course of subsequent RSV infection, appears to be caused by altered host immune response against RSV.

The lack of protective efficacy of FI-RSV is likely caused by one or more factors, including the development of poorly neutralizing antibodies against RSV-encoded epitopes, perhaps because of:

Denaturation of such epitopes
Incomplete affinity maturation of anti-RSV antibodies
Lack of a robust anti-RSV CTL response as shown in animal studies[24–26]

The potentiation phenomenon appears to be caused by a vaccine-induced priming and delayed hypersensitivity response involving Th2 CD4+ T-cells.[26] It should be noted that a clinical trial using parenterally administered live virus also failed to provide protection, although enhanced RSV disease did not occur.[27]

Live-Attenuated/Genetically Engineered Respiratory Syncytial Virus Derivatives

The major goal of generating live-attenuated RSV strains is to create a vaccine with the capacity to elicit a broad, protective immune response without significant clinical illness. Such studies of live-attenuated RSV strains began with the isolation of RSV strains that were able to replicate better at less than 37°C (ie, at temperatures similar to those within the upper respiratory tract) than at 37°C (ie, within the lower respiratory tract), thereby reducing the risk of serious lower respiratory tract illness. To date, such strategies include:

Serial viral passages to identify and characterize cold-passaged (cp) strains
Chemical mutagenesis to generate mutant RSV strains with temperature-sensitive (ts) phenotypes
Reverse genetics to engineer recombinant RSV strains bearing attenuated phenotype while maintaining genetic stability[28]

Extensive serial passage at progressively lower temperatures led to the isolation of cpRSV, which remained replication-competent at 26°C.[29] Derivatives of cpRSV strains were generated by mutagenesis with 5-fluorouracil, and one such derivative, cpts248/404, was deemed sufficiently attenuated for clinical testing in RSV-naïve infants (1 to 2 months old).[30] In such a study, greater than 80% of infant subjects were infected by the attenuated RSV strain and had a greater than or equal to fourfold increase in RSV-specific IgA levels following challenge. Moreover, most vaccine recipients were resistant to infection by a second dose of the vaccine strain given 1 month after the primary challenge. Greater than 70% of 1- to 2-month-old infant vaccine recipients, however, developed nasal congestion at the time of peak viral titer. Thus, the phenotype of cpts248/404 strain was deemed as insufficiently attenuated for use in very young, RSV-naïve infants. The replication of this viral strain, however, appeared to be unrelated to the level of maternal antibodies among vaccine recipients, and there was no obvious evidence of vaccine-enhanced RSV disease in poststudy follow-up.

Another group of biologically derived RSV mutants was isolated from successive rounds of chemical mutagenesis of the group A strain RSS-2 and selection for ts phenotype. The final derivative, ts1C, was tested in intranasal challenge in a small study involving 22 healthy young adults.[31] Following such administration, 30% of vaccine recipients exhibited viral shedding, and among this subgroup, none demonstrated clinical signs and symptoms of respiratory diseases. Following intranasal challenge, nearly 70% exhibited a greater than or equal to twofold increase in serum titers of RSV-neutralizing antibodies, with the greater increases trending to correlate with lower prevaccination anti-RSV titers. Thus, this small-scale study provided support for increased study of this RSV strain in the adult population.

The advent of reverse genetics and elucidation of structure–function relationships for most RSV-encoded proteins has led to the generation and testing of second-generation live-attenuated vaccine candidates. To this end, the genomic RNA of live-attenuated RSV strains that were biologically derived or chemically mutagenized were sequenced to identify nucleotide changes potentially associated with the attenuated phenotype.[32-34] Such nucleotide changes (eg, mutation affecting aa1030 of the protein, have then been engineered into existing RSV strains in hopes of further attenuation. Deletions of RSV genes also have been attempted for further attenuation or for potentially increasing host response. For example, the deletion of the SH gene causes up to tenfold decrease in RSV replication in primates, while the deletion of NS1 or NS2 genes may increase the expression of type 1 interferon and thus potentially increase immunogenicity in vaccine recipients.[35,36]

Based on the previously mentioned genetic manipulations, at least two lineages of second-generation, live-attenuated RSV vaccine candidates have been generated. The first is rA2cp248/404/1030ΔSH, in which the cp248/404 was engineered to bear the L protein aa1030 mutation and the deletion of the SH gene.[32] When evaluated in RSV-naïve, very young infants (1 to 2 months old), a greater than or equal to fourfold increase in anti-RSV antibodies was noted in 44% of infants previously uninfected with RSV. The second dose of the vaccine strain given within 2 months of the priming dose was restricted significantly, indicating that protective immunity was achieved in most RSV-naïve vaccine recipients.[37] The rA2cp248/404/1030ΔSH strain, however, appears to exhibit some degree of genetic and phenotypic instability during replication, likely necessitating further manipulations for additional vaccine testing.[37] The second line of reverse genetics-mediated RSV vaccine candidate is comprised of A2cp derivative bearing deletions in the NS2 gene (ie, rA2cpΔNS2, rA2cp530/1009ΔNS2, and rA2cp248/404ΔNS2).[38] In limited clinical studies, the first of the three strains appeared to be overly attenuated in adults, while the latter two were overattenuated for use in the pediatric population.[38] Thus, derivatives of RSV strains deleted for NS2 are being studied for additional genetic manipulations designed to achieve a compromise between over- and underattenuated phenotype.

Taken together, the live-attenuated RSV vaccine approach has shown promise based on current knowledge of cp/ts mutations within the genome, essential/nonessential RSV genes, and structure/function of RSV-encoded genes. The major challenge to this approach remains the need of achieving an appropriate balance between the two priorities of live-attenuated RSV vaccine development (overattenuation/suboptimal immunogenicity and underattenuation/bearing pathogenic potential).[19]

Subunit Vaccines

RSV-derived F and G proteins and their derivatives bearing neutralizing epitopes have undergone preclinical and clinical assessments as nonreplicating protein subunit vaccines. The first of such preclinical studies used RSV F and G proteins that were purified from RSV-infected cell cultures and F and F/G chimeric proteins produced in baculovirus-infected insect cells or transfected mammalian cell lines[39,40] Rodents immunized with these preparations generated antibodies similar to those observed for FI-RSV in that despite recognition of RSV antigen in ELISAs, the resulting antibodies were poorly neutralizing.[17,41] In addition, rodents immunized with such RSV-encoded proteins and subsequently challenged 3 to 6 months later developed lung pathologies similar to those observed for FI-RSV.[17] To circumvent the potential deleterious consequences of subunit vaccination, several groups have used various adjuvants, including those specific for various toll-like receptors (TLRs) (eg, monophosphoryl lipid A [MPL] for TLR-4, CpG oligonucleotides for [TLR-9]) and have reported that in some cases, the use of adjuvants can significantly alter the immunogenicity and adverse effects of subunit vaccines.[42,43] Of relevance is the recent observation that TLR agonists may play a significant role in the affinity maturation of antibodies against RSV-encoded proteins.[44] Thus, in principle, appropriate TLR stimulation during vaccination with RSV subunit preparations may generate high-affinity anti-RSV antibodies that recognize appropriate epitopes in nondenatured configurations.

With respect to clinical evaluation of RSV subunit vaccine candidates, several preparations of RSV-encoded proteins have been tested. Such preparations include: PFP (purified F protein) derivatives (PFP-1, -2, and -3); FG chimeric protein; a copurified formulation of F, G, and M proteins, and a bacterially derived RSV G derivative (BBG2Na). Such efforts are described here briefly.

The PFP series have been purified from RSV-infected Vero cells, and successive versions are comprised of higher purity of RSV F (ie, 90% to 95% F for PFP-1 versus greater than 98% for PFP-2 and -3).[45,46] PFP-1 has been tested in RSV-seropositive children in two clinical trials involving RSV-seropositive children 24 to 48 months old and 18 to 36 months old.[46,47] In these studies, no obvious adverse events were evident and a greater than or equal to fourfold increase in RSV-neutralizing antibody titer was observed in most subjects. A single priming intramuscular dose of PFP-2 (50 μg) was administered to 1- to 12-year-old children with bronchopulmonary dysplasia (n = 10) or 1 to 8 year olds with cystic fibrosis (n = 17). In this study, most participants exhibited a greater than or equal to fourfold increase in RSV-neutralizing antibody titers.[48,49] PFP-3 has been tested as a single 30 μg intramuscular vaccination dose in a phase 2 study among 143 1- to 12-year-old children with cystic fibrosis.[50] As in the case of PFP-2, PFP-3 also elicited a greater than or equal to fourfold increase in RSV neutralizing titers. The rate of RSV infection after vaccination, however, was not significantly different between the vaccinated and control groups. In two studies involving elderly adults, a single 50 μg dose of PFP-2 was also immunogenic in 61% (out of 33 subjects older than 60 years) and 47% (of 36 frail elderly adults older than 65 years).[51] Lastly, a single 20 μg dose of PFP-2 administered to 20 pregnant women was tolerated well.[52] Although the vaccine led to a greater than or equal to fourfold increase in anti-F antibodies in most vaccine recipients and their infants up to 6 months following birth, only 10% of the study subjects had a corresponding greater than or equal to fourfold increase in RSV-neutralizing antibody titers.

BBG2Na, a bacterially derived protein bearing aa130–230 of subgroup A RSV G protein fused to the albumin-binding domain of streptococcal protein G, also has undergone preclinical and clinical evaluation. In rodent models, BBG2Na conferred protection against RSV even though it generated modest levels of RSV-neutralizing antibodies.[53] In limited primate studies, however, this antigen was associated with limited viral challenge protection and also with Th2-biased immune response.[54] Among healthy young adults and elderly adults, this antigen also was tolerated well in phase 2 studies.[19] In a phase 3 study involving elderly adults, however, anti-RSV serum antibody titers declined significantly within 4 weeks after vaccination, and a limited number of unanticipated adverse events has been reported.

With respect to other clinical trials with RSV subunit/protein-derived vaccine candidates, limited data are available. For FG chimeric protein testing, phase 1 and 2 studies involving its administration with various adjuvants have been started but not reported formally.[19] In one study, a copurified formulation of RSV F, G, and M proteins were emulsified in one of two adjuvants (aluminum hydroxide and poly(di[carboxylato-phenoxy]phosphazene; PCPP)) and administered to healthy adults (total n = 70).[55] In this study, both vaccine formulations induced similar levels of greater than or equal to fourfold increase in RSV-neutralizing antibody titers and collectively in greater than 80% of the study population. In a large-scale phase 2 study of 1169 elderly adults who had cardiopulmonary conditions, the RSV F, G and M-containing vaccine was immunogenic. A greater proportion of subjects immunized with nonadjuvanted vaccine had a greater than or equal to fourfold increase in RSV neutralizing antibody ters as compared with titers in the group challenged with alum-containing vaccine candidate (168 of 383 [44%] versus 129 of 400 [33%]).[56]

Short peptides derived from RSV F and G proteins have been tested in animal models. In the case of short, RSV F-derived peptides, limited immunogenicity was seen.[57] Recent data suggest that in mice, administration of bacterially derived short fragments of RSV F (including aa255–278 and 412–524) fused to the ctxA(2)B cholera holotoxin led to anti-F, RSV-neutralizing antibody response and a modest protective efficacy in mouse RSV challenge studies.[58,59] For RSV G, the aa sequence (174–187) derived from the central core of RSV G has been administered to mice; in such experiments, protections against RSV infection was noted despite inefficient RSV-neutralizing response.[60,61]

An alternative platform for RSV subunit vaccines is virus-like particles (VLPs), which are nonreplicating, noninfectious particles derived from virus-encoded proteins.[62] In the case of human papillomavirus (HPV) VLP-based licensed vaccine, the HPV L1 capsid protein self-assembles into particles that appear morphologically indistinguishable from native HPV virions.[63] The resulting VLPs elicit strong humoral and cellular immune responses and provide durable protection against HPV. Other virus-encoded proteins, such as the influenza hemaglutinin and the hepatitis B surface antigen (HBSAg), also can form VLPs, and in the latter case, they have been engineered to contain an RSV-encoded CTL epitope.[64] Most recently, nanoparticles derived from bacterially derived RSV nucleocapsid proteins have been shown to confer a moderate degree of protection against RSV challenge in rodent models.[65] Because of their potent immunogenicity, VLPs may be an alternative platform for RSV subunit vaccine, provided that appropriate epitopes can be presented successfully.

Vector-based Respiratory Syncytial Virus Vaccines

Several live virus vectors have been generated to express RSV-encoded proteins. Such vectors have included vaccinia virus (mouse-adapted WR strain and the MVA strain), engineered to express RSV F and G, and adenovirus derivatives expressing RSV F.[66,67] In these cases, there was no significant immunogenicity or protective efficacy in primates.[68–70] More recently, genetically engineered varieties of parainfluenza viruses including human parainfluenza virus (HPIV3), Sendai virus (SeV), and a chimeric bovine parainfluenza virus (BPIV)/HPIV3 have been used to express RSV F and G under the control of endogenous parainfluenza virus (PIV) gene expression signals. These have the possibility of being developed as a bivalent RSV/PIV vaccine for children.[71–74] B/PIV3-expressing RSV F has been shown to be immunogenic and efficacious in RSV protective challenge studies in primates and is being evaluated in clinical studies.[75]

Recent studies have described various strategies to express RSV F or G in the context of live bacterial vectors and nonreplicating viral vectors. For example, *Staphylococcus carnosus*, a nonpathogenic bacterium, has been modified to express on its surface three portions of the RSV G protein fused to a fragment of the cholera B subunit protein.[76] The resulting bacteria have the potential advantage of oral or intranasal administration, but they were found to provide limited and variable protective efficacy in mouse RSV challenge studies. RSV F or G has been expressed in the context on replication-incompetent (ie, replicon-based) alphavirus vectors, and the avian Newcastle disease virus and human rhinovirus type 14.[77–80] Most of these viral-vectored RSV vaccine candidates are immunogenic and protective to varying degrees in mouse RSV challenge studies.

DNA Vaccines

Through various routes, including intramuscular, intradermal, microparticle gene gun, or DNA-carbohydrate/albumin intranasal approaches, immunization of rodents with DNA plasmids encoding RSV F or G proteins has shown that administration of DNA is immunogenic and protective to a limited degree in RSV challenge experiments.[81–84] DNA-based RSV vaccine has the potential to express RSV-encoded proteins in its native structure, and may do so in the context of the immature immune system in infants, thereby overcoming the maternal antibody-associated immunosuppression of anti-RSV response. Lingering technical challenges for this approach include: the time of onset of immune response, the amount of DNA required to generate a clinically relevant immune response, and the likely need for multiple repeated administration of such DNA molecules.

SUMMARY

RSV vaccine development remains a high priority based on the burden of diseases and limited number of licensed prophylactic and therapeutic options. Previous and current efforts involve the development and preclinical/clinical (where appropriate) testing of live-attenuated RSV strains, RSV subunit-based proteins, live/nonreplicating vector-derived vaccine candidates, and DNA-based approaches. Based on the historical experience with formalin-inactivated RSV vaccine, further studies on RSV vaccine development likely will require continued safety and efficacy monitoring. Because immune response against RSV following natural infection is incomplete, it is possible that two vaccines—one for pediatric, RSV-naïve subjects and another for RSV-infected elderly adults—will be developed.

REFERENCES

1. Hall CB, McCarthy CA. Respiratory syncytial virus. In: Mandell GL, Bennett JE, Dolin R, editors. Principles and practices of infectious disease, vol. 6. Philadelphia: Elsevier Churchill Livingstone; 2004. p. 2008–26.
2. Hall CB, Walsh EE, Long CE, et al. Immunity to and frequency of reinfection with respiratory syncytial virus. J Infect Dis 1991;163:693–8.
3. Thompson WW, Shay DK, Weintraub E, et al. Mortality associated with influenza and respiratory syncytial virus in the United States. JAMA 2003;289:179–86.
4. Falsey AR, Hennessey PA, Formica MA, et al. Respiratory syncytial virus infection in elderly and high-risk adults. N Engl J Med 2005;352:1749–59.
5. Collins PL, Graham BS. Viral and host factors in human respiratory syncytial virus pathogenesis. J Virol 2008;82:2040–55.
6. Taylor G, Stott EJ, Bew M, et al. Monoclonal antibodies protect against respiratory syncytial virus. Lancet 1983;2:976.
7. Walsh EE, Schlesinger JJ, Brandriss MW. Protection from respiratory syncytial virus infection in cotton rats by passive transfer of monoclonal antibodies. Infect Immun 1984;43:756–8.
8. Walsh EE, Cote PJ, Fernie BF, et al. Analysis of the respiratory syncytial virus fusion protein using monoclonal and polyclonal antibodies. J Gen Virol 1986; 67:505–13.
9. Palivizumab, a humanized respiratory syncytial virus monoclonal antibody, reduces hospitalization from respiratory syncytial virus infection in high-risk infants. IMpact-RSV Study Group. Pediatrics 1998;102:531–7.

0. Zhang L, Peeples ME, Boucher RC, et al. Respiratory syncytial virus infection of human airway epithelial cells is polarized, specific to ciliated cells, and without obvious cytopathology. J Virol 2002;76:5654–66.
1. Openshaw PJ, Tregoning JS. Immune responses and disease enhancement during respiratory syncytial virus infection. Clin Microbiol Rev 2005;18:541–55.
2. Braciale TJ. Respiratory syncytial virus and T cells: interplay between the virus and the host adaptive immune system. Proc Am Thorac Soc 2005;2:141–6.
3. Graham BS, Bunton LA, Wright PF, et al. Role of T lymphocyte subsets in the pathogenesis of primary infection and rechallenge with respiratory syncytial virus in mice. J Clin Invest 1991;88:1026–33.
4. Alwan WH, Record FM, Openshaw PJ. CD4+ T cells clear virus but augment disease in mice infected with respiratory syncytial virus. Comparison with the effects of CD8+ T cells. Clin Exp Immunol 1992;88:527–36.
5. Tang YW, Graham BS. T cell source of type 1 cytokines determines illness patterns in respiratory syncytial virus-infected mice. J Clin Invest 1997;99: 2183–91.
6. Peebles RS Jr, Graham BS. Pathogenesis of respiratory syncytial virus infection in the murine model. Proc Am Thorac Soc 2005;2:110–5.
17. Murphy BR, Sotnikov AV, Lawrence LA, et al. Enhanced pulmonary histopathology is observed in cotton rats immunized with formalin-inactivated respiratory syncytial virus (RSV) or purified F glycoprotein and challenged with RSV 3–6 months after immunization. Vaccine 1990;8:497–502.
18. Openshaw PJ, Clarke SL, Record FM. Pulmonary eosinophilic response to respiratory syncytial virus infection in mice sensitized to the major surface glycoprotein G. Int Immunol 1992;4:493–500.
19. Collins PL, Murphy BR. Vaccines against human respiratory syncytial virus. In: Cane PA, editor. Respiratory syncytial virus. Amsterdam: Elsevier; 2007. p. 233–77.
20. Fulginiti VA, Eller JJ, Sieber OF, et al. Respiratory virus immunization. I. A field trial of two inactivated respiratory virus vaccines: an aqueous trivalent parainfluenza virus vaccine and an alum-precipitated respiratory syncytial virus vaccine. Am J Epidemiol 1969;89:435–48.
21. Kapikian AZ, Mitchell RH, Chanock RM, et al. An epidemiologic study of altered clinical reactivity to respiratory syncytial (RS) virus infection in children previously vaccinated with an inactivated RS virus vaccine. Am J Epidemiol 1969;89:405–21.
22. Chin J, Magoffin RL, Shearer LA, et al. Field evaluation of a respiratory syncytial virus vaccine and a trivalent parainfluenza virus vaccine in a pediatric population. Am J Epidemiol 1969;89:449–63.
23. Kim HW, Canchola JG, Brandt CD, et al. Respiratory syncytial virus disease in infants despite prior administration of antigenic inactivated vaccine. Am J Epidemiol 1969;89:422–34.
24. Murphy BR, Walsh EE. Formalin-inactivated respiratory syncytial virus vaccine induces antibodies to the fusion glycoprotein that are deficient in fusion-inhibiting activity. J Clin Microbiol 1988;26:1595–7.
25. Peebles RS Jr, Sheller JR, Collins RD, et al. Respiratory syncytial virus (RSV)-induced airway hyper-responsiveness in allergically sensitized mice is inhibited by live RSV and exacerbated by formalin-inactivated RSV. J Infect Dis 2000; 182:671–7.
26. Prince GA, Jenson AB, Hemming VG, et al. Enhancement of respiratory syncytial virus pulmonary pathology in cotton rats by prior intramuscular inoculation of formalin-inactivated virus. J Virol 1986;57:721–8.

27. Belshe RB, Van Voris LP, Mufson MA. Parenteral administration of live respiratory syncytial virus vaccine: results of a field trial. J Infect Dis 1982;145:311–9.

28. Collins PL, Murphy BR. New generation live vaccines against human respiratory syncytial virus designed by reverse genetics. Proc Am Thorac Soc 2005;2:166–73

29. Friedwald W, Forsyth B, Smith C, et al. Low-temperature grown RS virus in adult volunteers. JAMA 1968;204:142–6.

30. Wright PF, Karron RA, Belshe RB, et al. Evaluation of a live, cold-passaged temperature-sensitive, respiratory syncytial virus vaccine candidate in infancy J Infect Dis 2000;182:1331–42.

31. Pringle CR, Filipiuk AH, Robinson BS, et al. Immunogenicity and pathogenicity of a triple temperature-sensitive modified respiratory syncytial virus in adult volunteers. Vaccine 1993;11:473–8.

32. Whitehead SS, Firestone CY, Karron RA, et al. Addition of a missense mutation present in the L gene of respiratory syncytial virus (RSV) cpts530/1030 to RSV vaccine candidate cpts248/404 increases its attenuation and temperature sensitivity. J Virol 1999;73:871–7.

33. Whitehead SS, Firestone CY, Collins PL, et al. A single nucleotide substitution in the transcription start signal of the M2 gene of respiratory syncytial virus vaccine candidate cpts248/404 is the major determinant of the temperature-sensitive and attenuation phenotypes. Virology 1998;247:232–9.

34. Juhasz K, Whitehead SS, Boulanger CA, et al. The two amino acid substitutions in the L protein of cpts530/1009, a live-attenuated respiratory syncytial virus candidate vaccine, are independent temperature-sensitive, and attenuation mutations. Vaccine 1999;17:1416–24.

35. Whitehead SS, Juhasz K, Firestone CY, et al. Recombinant respiratory syncytial virus (RSV) bearing a set of mutations from cold-passaged RSV is attenuated in chimpanzees. J Virol 1998;72:4467–71.

36. Teng MN, Whitehead SS, Bermingham A, et al. Recombinant respiratory syncytial virus that does not express the NS1 or M2-2 protein is highly attenuated and immunogenic in chimpanzees. J Virol 2000;74:9317–21.

37. Karron RA, Wright PF, Belshe RB, et al. Identification of a recombinant live attenuated respiratory syncytial virus vaccine candidate that is highly attenuated in infants. J Infect Dis 2005;191:1093–104.

38. Wright PF, Karron RA, Madhi SA, et al. The interferon antagonist NS2 protein of respiratory syncytial virus is an important virulence determinant for humans. J Infect Dis 2006;193:573–81.

39. Walsh EE, Hall CB, Briselli M, et al. Immunization with glycoprotein subunits of respiratory syncytial virus to protect cotton rats against viral infection. J Infect Dis 1987;155:1198–204.

40. Wathen MW, Kakuk TJ, Brideau RJ, et al. Vaccination of cotton rats with a chimeric FG glycoprotein of human respiratory syncytial virus induces minimal pulmonary pathology on challenge. J Infect Dis 1991;163:477–82.

41. Murphy BR, Sotnikov A, Paradiso PR, et al. Immunization of cotton rats with the fusion (F) and large (G) glycoproteins of respiratory syncytial virus (RSV) protects against RSV challenge without potentiating RSV disease. Vaccine 1989;7:533–40.

42. Hancock GE, Heers KM, Pryharski KS, et al. Adjuvants recognized by toll-like receptors inhibit the induction of polarized type 2 T cell responses by natural attachment (G) protein of respiratory syncytial virus. Vaccine 2003;21:4348–58.

43. Prince GA, Denamur F, Deschamps M, et al. Monophosphoryl lipid A adjuvant reverses a principal histologic parameter of formalin-inactivated respiratory syncytial virus vaccine-induced disease. Vaccine 2001;19:2048–54.

4. Delgado MF, Coviello S, Monsalvo AC, et al. Lack of antibody affinity maturation due to poor toll-like receptor stimulation leads to enhanced respiratory syncytial virus disease. Nat Med 2009;15:34–41.

5. Belshe RB, Anderson EL, Walsh EE. Immunogenicity of purified F glycoprotein of respiratory syncytial virus: clinical and immune responses to subsequent natural infection in children. J Infect Dis 1993;168:1024–9.

46. Tristram DA, Welliver RC, Mohar CK, et al. Immunogenicity and safety of respiratory syncytial virus subunit vaccine in seropositive children 18–36 months old. J Infect Dis 1993;167:191–5.

47. Paradiso PR, Hildreth SW, Hogerman DA, et al. Safety and immunogenicity of a subunit respiratory syncytial virus vaccine in children 24 to 48 months old. Pediatr Infect Dis J 1994;13:792–8.

48. Piedra PA, Grace S, Jewell A, et al. Purified fusion protein vaccine protects against lower respiratory tract illness during respiratory syncytial virus season in children with cystic fibrosis. Pediatr Infect Dis J 1996;15:23–31.

49. Groothuis JR, King SJ, Hogerman DA, et al. Safety and immunogenicity of a purified F protein respiratory syncytial virus (PFP-2) vaccine in seropositive children with bronchopulmonary dysplasia. J Infect Dis 1998;177:467–9.

50. Piedra PA, Cron SG, Jewell A, et al. Immunogenicity of a new purified fusion protein vaccine to respiratory syncytial virus: a multicenter trial in children with cystic fibrosis. Vaccine 2003;21:2448–60.

51. Falsey AR, Walsh EE. Safety and immunogenicity of a respiratory syncytial virus subunit vaccine (PFP-2) in ambulatory adults over age 60. Vaccine 1996;14:1214–8.

52. Munoz FM, Piedra PA, Glezen WP. Safety and immunogenicity of respiratory syncytial virus purified fusion protein-2 vaccine in pregnant women. Vaccine 2003;21:3465–7.

53. Power UF, Plotnicky-Gilquin H, Huss T, et al. Induction of protective immunity in rodents by vaccination with a prokaryotically expressed recombinant fusion protein containing a respiratory syncytial virus G protein fragment. Virology 1997;230:155–66.

54. de Waal L, Power UF, Yuksel S, et al. Evaluation of BBG2Na in infant macaques: specific immune responses after vaccination and RSV challenge. Vaccine 2004;22:915–22.

55. Ison MG, Mills J, Openshaw P, et al. Current research on respiratory viral infections: fourth international symposium. Antiviral Res 2002;55:227–78.

56. Falsey AR, Walsh EE, Capellan J, et al. Comparison of the safety and immunogenicity of 2 respiratory syncytial virus (RSV) vaccines—nonadjuvanted vaccine or vaccine adjuvanted with alum—given concomitantly with influenza vaccine to high-risk elderly individuals. J Infect Dis 2008;198:1317–26.

57. Trudel M, Stott EJ, Taylor G, et al. Synthetic peptides corresponding to the F protein of RSV stimulate murine B and T cells but fail to confer protection. Arch Virol 1991;117:59–71.

58. Singh SR, Dennis VA, Carter CL, et al. Respiratory syncytial virus recombinant F protein (residues 255-278) induces a helper T cell type 1 immune response in mice. Viral Immunol 2007;20:261–75.

59. Singh SR, Dennis VA, Carter CL, et al. Immunogenicity and efficacy of recombinant RSV-F vaccine in a mouse model. Vaccine 2007;25:6211–23.

60. Trudel M, Nadon F, Seguin C, et al. Protection of BALB/c mice from respiratory syncytial virus infection by immunization with a synthetic peptide derived from the G-glycoprotein. Virology 1991;185:749–57.

61. Bastien N, Trudel M, Simard C. Complete protection of mice from respiratory syncytial virus infection following mucosal delivery of synthetic peptide vaccines. Vaccine 1999;17:832–6.
62. Jennings GT, Bachmann MF. The coming of age of virus-like particle vaccines. Biol Chem 2008;389:521–36.
63. Siddiqui MA, Perry CM. Human papillomavirus quadrivalent (types 6, 11, 16, 18) recombinant vaccine (Gardasil). Drugs 2006;66:1263–71 [discussion: 1272–3].
64. Woo WP, Doan T, Herd KA, et al. Hepatitis B surface antigen vector delivers protective cytotoxic T-lymphocyte responses to disease-relevant foreign epitopes. J Virol 2006;80:3975–84.
65. Roux X, Dubuquoy C, Durand G, et al. Subnucleocapsid nanoparticles: a nasal vaccine against respiratory syncytial virus. PLoS One 2008;3:e1766.
66. Connors M, Collins PL, Firestone CY, et al. Respiratory syncytial virus (RSV) F, G, M2 (22K), and N proteins each induce resistance to RSV challenge, but resistance induced by M2 and N proteins is relatively short-lived. J Virol 1991;65:1634–7.
67. Wyatt LS, Whitehead SS, Venanzi KA, et al. Priming and boosting immunity to respiratory syncytial virus by recombinant replication-defective vaccinia virus MVA. Vaccine 1999;18:392–7.
68. Collins PL, Purcell RH, London WT, et al. Evaluation in chimpanzees of vaccinia virus recombinants that express the surface glycoproteins of human respiratory syncytial virus. Vaccine 1990;8:164–8.
69. Crowe JE Jr, Collins PL, London WT, et al. A comparison in chimpanzees of the immunogenicity and efficacy of live attenuated respiratory syncytial virus (RSV) temperature-sensitive mutant vaccines and vaccinia virus recombinants that express the surface glycoproteins of RSV. Vaccine 1993;11:1395–404.
70. de Waal L, Wyatt LS, Yuksel S, et al. Vaccination of infant macaques with a recombinant modified vaccinia virus ankara expressing the respiratory syncytial virus F and G genes does not predispose for immunopathology. Vaccine 2004;22:923–6.
71. Takimoto T, Hurwitz JL, Zhan X, et al. Recombinant sendai virus as a novel vaccine candidate for respiratory syncytial virus. Viral Immunol 2005;18:255–66.
72. Tang RS, Schickli JH, MacPhail M, et al. Effects of human metapneumovirus and respiratory syncytial virus antigen insertion in two 3′ proximal genome positions of bovine/human parainfluenza virus type 3 on virus replication and immunogenicity. J Virol 2003;77:10819–28.
73. Schmidt AC, McAuliffe JM, Murphy BR, et al. Recombinant bovine/human parainfluenza virus type 3 (B/HPIV3) expressing the respiratory syncytial virus (RSV) G and F proteins can be used to achieve simultaneous mucosal immunization against RSV and HPIV3. J Virol 2001;75:4594–603.
74. Schmidt AC, Wenzke DR, McAuliffe JM, et al. Mucosal immunization of rhesus monkeys against respiratory syncytial virus subgroups A and B and human parainfluenza virus type 3 by using a live cDNA-derived vaccine based on a host range-attenuated bovine parainfluenza virus type 3 vector backbone. J Virol 2002;76:1089–99.
75. Tang RS, MacPhail M, Schickli JH, et al. Parainfluenza virus type 3 expressing the native or soluble fusion (F) protein of respiratory syncytial virus (RSV) confers protection from RSV infection in African green monkeys. J Virol 2004;78:11198–207.
76. Cano F, Plotnicky-Gilquin H, Nguyen TN, et al. Partial protection to respiratory syncytial virus (RSV) elicited in mice by intranasal immunization using live staphylococci with surface-displayed RSV-peptides. Vaccine 2000;18:2743–52.

7. Mok H, Lee S, Utley TJ, et al. Venezuelan equine encephalitis virus replicon particles encoding respiratory syncytial virus surface glycoproteins induce protective mucosal responses in mice and cotton rats. J Virol 2007;81:13710–22.

8. Elliott MB, Chen T, Terio NB, et al. Alphavirus replicon particles encoding the fusion or attachment glycoproteins of respiratory syncytial virus elicit protective immune responses in BALB/c mice and functional serum antibodies in rhesus macaques. Vaccine 2007;25:7132–44.

9. Martinez-Sobrido L, Gitiban N, Fernandez-Sesma A, et al. Protection against respiratory syncytial virus by a recombinant Newcastle disease virus vector. J Virol 2006;80:1130–9.

10. Dollenmaier G, Mosier SM, Scholle F, et al. Membrane-associated respiratory syncytial virus F protein expressed from a human rhinovirus type 14 vector is immunogenic. Virology 2001;281:216–30.

11. Li X, Sambhara S, Li CX, et al. Protection against respiratory syncytial virus infection by DNA immunization. J Exp Med 1998;188:681–8.

12. Li X, Sambhara S, Li CX, et al. Plasmid DNA encoding the respiratory syncytial virus G protein is a promising vaccine candidate. Virology 2000;269:54–65.

13. Kumar M, Behera AK, Lockey RF, et al. Intranasal gene transfer by chitosan-DNA nanospheres protects BALB/c mice against acute respiratory syncytial virus infection. Hum Gene Ther 2002;13:1415–25.

14. Bembridge GP, Rodriguez N, Garcia-Beato R, et al. Respiratory syncytial virus infection of gene gun vaccinated mice induces Th2-driven pulmonary eosinophilia even in the absence of sensitisation to the fusion (F) or attachment (G) protein. Vaccine 2000;19:1038–46.

Respiratory Viruses in Bronchiolitis and Their Link to Recurrent Wheezing and Asthma

Jonathan M. Mansbach, MD[a],*, Carlos A. Camargo, Jr, MD, DrPH[b]

KEYWORDS

- Bronchiolitis • Asthma • Respiratory syncytial virus
- Rhinovirus • Wheezing • Vitamin D

One of the earliest and most common infectious respiratory conditions of childhood is bronchiolitis.[1,2] A child who has severe bronchiolitis (eg, an episode requiring hospitalization) is at increased risk for recurrent wheezing of childhood and eventual asthma.[3–5] Estimates vary but approximately 80% to 90% of asthma begins before age 6 years, with 70% of children who have asthma having asthmalike symptoms before age 3 years.[6,7] Although many environmental and genetic factors may play a role in the pathway from bronchiolitis to asthma,[3,8] this article focuses on the viruses that have been linked to bronchiolitis and how these viruses may predict or contribute to future wheezing and asthma. The article also discusses vitamin D as an emerging risk factor for respiratory infections and wheezing.

DEFINITIONS OF LOWER RESPIRATORY TRACT INFECTION

In the United States, lower respiratory tract infections (LRTI) represent almost 60% of infant infectious disease hospitalizations[9] and bronchiolitis is the most common LRTI.[10] Despite its high frequency, bronchiolitis remains a clinical diagnosis[11–13] without a common international definition.[10,14–18] In 2006, the American Academy of Pediatrics defined bronchiolitis as a child younger than 2 years of age who has

This work was supported by grants K23 AI-77801 and U01 AI-67693 from the National Institutes of Health (Bethesda, MD) and the Massachusetts General Hospital Center for D-receptor Activation Research (Boston, MA).
[a] Department of Medicine, Children's Hospital Boston, Harvard Medical School, Main Clinical Building 9 South, #9157, Boston, MA 02115, USA
[b] Department of Emergency Medicine, Division of Rheumatology, Allergy, and Immunology, Massachusetts General Hospital, Harvard Medical School, 326 Cambridge Street, Suite 410, Boston, MA 02114, USA
* Corresponding author.
E-mail address: jonathan.mansbach@childrens.harvard.edu (J.M. Mansbach).

"rhinitis, tachypnea, wheezing, cough, crackles, use of accessory muscles, and/or nasal flaring."[10] This definition is broad, and when children younger than 2 years of age present to care with symptoms suggestive of an LRTI, they receive various diagnostic labels, such as bronchiolitis, wheezing, cough, reactive airways disease, asthma, or pneumonia.[19]

As our understanding of LRTI evolves and we identify more clearly the risk factors for children developing recurrent wheezing in preschool years (and asthma as they grow older), we may need to adjust our LRTI definitions. Indeed, based on 259 wheezing hospitalized children aged 3 to 35 months participating in a systemic corticosteroid and wheezing study in Finland, Jartti and colleagues[18] recently suggested that the diagnosis of bronchiolitis should be restricted either to children younger than 24 months of age who have their first episode of wheezing or to children younger than 12 months of age.

BRONCHIOLITIS EPIDEMIOLOGY

With its broad definition, bronchiolitis is the leading cause of hospitalization for infants in the United States[20,21] and the associated hospitalization costs are more than $500 million per year.[22] In a nationally representative sample, bronchiolitis hospitalization rates increased 2.4-fold from 1980 to 1996[20] and in a Tennessee Medicaid database there was a 41% increase in bronchiolitis visits at all levels of care (ie, inpatient, emergency department [ED], and outpatient clinic) from 1996 to 2003.[2]

BRONCHIOLITIS PATHOGENS

Respiratory syncytial virus (RSV) is the most common pathogen associated with bronchiolitis.[1,23] Although most children are infected with RSV by age 2 years,[24,25] relatively few children (<40%) develop clinically recognized bronchiolitis.[24,26] Among those children who develop bronchiolitis, most have a mild course; approximately 2% to 3% will be hospitalized[20,27] and less than 1% will be admitted to an ICU, intubated, or die.[28–31]

Other viruses that have been linked to bronchiolitis include rhinovirus (RV),[32,33] human metapneumovirus (hMPV),[34] influenza A/B,[35,36] parainfluenza (PIV),[37] and adenovirus.[38,39] Coronaviruses also have been linked to lower respiratory tract disease in children,[40] including the strains NL-63[41] or New Haven[42] and HKU1.[43–45] More recently discovered viruses include human bocavirus[46–49] and the polyomaviruses WU[50] and KI.[51] The clinical relevance of these two polyomaviruses is uncertain.[52] Furthermore, there is conflicting literature about the relevance of bacterial coinfection in children who have viral bronchiolitis, especially those children requiring intensive care.[53–56]

Although myriad infectious causes are associated with bronchiolitis, it remains unclear if the viral cause of a child's bronchiolitis illness is clinically relevant for either the short- or long-term care of the individual child. For short-term care, knowing the infectious cause identifies children who have influenza who may benefit from oseltamivir; it also helps cohort hospitalized children. Otherwise the current consensus is that knowledge of the viral etiology—among those viruses with easily accessible point-of-care testing (eg, RSV and influenza)—does not affect treatment of the individual patient.[10] As rapid microarray testing becomes less costly and more widely used, however, we are likely to learn much more about the short- and long-term implications of the diverse viruses linked to bronchiolitis. Indeed, these new data could markedly change current understanding and consensus.

EPIDEMIOLOGY OF PATHOGENS AT DIFFERENT LEVELS OF CARE

Several studies have examined the epidemiology of different viruses associated with RTI in hospitalized children,[33,37,57-61] but there are fewer studies investigating the epidemiology of viruses linked to bronchiolitis in children presenting to the ED or in outpatient clinics.[62-65] In this section, we present one representative study from the three levels of care (inpatient, ED, outpatient clinic) from different regions of the world.

An inpatient study by Wolf and colleagues[66] compared the clinical features of RSV, hMPV, influenza A, parainfluenza, and adenovirus in 516 Israeli children younger than 2 years of age who were hospitalized with LRTI over a 1-year period. The investigators detected a virus in 57% of the children tested in this single-center study. Children hospitalized with RSV were younger than those hospitalized with hMPV, but the severity of the respiratory illness caused by RSV and hMPV was similar and higher than that of influenza A.

In a multicenter ED-based study of 277 United States children who had physician-diagnosed bronchiolitis,[67] we examined the frequencies of RSV, RV, hMPV, and influenza A/B during one bronchiolitis winter season. We detected a virus in 84% of the samples; RSV was the most common (64%) and RV the second most common (16%).

In a community-based birth cohort sample of Australian children at high risk for atopy (ie, one parent with history of asthma, hay fever, or eczema), Kusel and colleagues[68] examined the frequency of nine different pathogens in these children during their first year. When the children had acute respiratory infections (either upper or lower) the children had nasopharyngeal samples taken. For upper and lower respiratory tract infections in the first year of life, RV was the most frequent cause (48%) and RSV the second most common (11%).

Most data indicate that RSV and RV are the two most common viruses associated with LRTI in early childhood. RSV is detected more frequently from children in the hospital or ED and RV is detected more frequently from children in the outpatient clinic setting.

COINFECTIONS

When considering the cohorting of inpatients, it is important to realize that the aforementioned infectious agents may cause bronchiolitis in isolation or in combination with other infectious agents. Although older studies report coinfections (eg, detection of two or more viruses from the same biologic sample) in 4.4% to 23.7% of children younger than 3 years of age who had respiratory illnesses,[69-74] recent studies have found 20% to 27% coinfections when testing hospitalized children who had LRTI.[59,61] There is a lack of clear data, however, about the clinical characteristics of children who have coinfections. Some studies have found no increase in the severity of disease from coinfections as measured by hospital length of stay,[75] clinical symptoms,[70,71] a severity score,[76] or duration of illness.[72] Other data, however, demonstrate that children infected with multiple pathogens have more severe bronchiolitis as measured by higher hospitalization rates[77] or degree of hypoxia and longer hospital length of stay.[61]

It is likely that the clinical course of coinfections will differ; some combinations of viruses are more or less deleterious than others. One combination that is believed to increase the severity of illness is RSV and hMPV coinfection.[78] As part of a larger study examining severe bronchiolitis, RSV and hMPV were identified in the bronchoalveolar fluid of 70% of 30 intubated infants.[79] In a different study, 72% of 25 intubated children had RSV and hMPV coinfection compared with 10% of 171 children hospitalized on the general wards.[80] Interestingly, hMPV was also found in 5 of 9 patients during the 2003 severe acute respiratory syndrome or SARS outbreak in Canada.[8] Recent studies investigating RSV and hMPV suggest that they may have distinctive pathogenesis,[66] elicit unique cytokine profiles,[82–85] and use different mechanisms to activate human dendritic cells, which play a key role in the adaptive immune response.[86] Moreover, a prospective study by Laham and colleagues[87] measured cytokine levels in Buenos Aires infants presenting with upper or lower respiratory tract illness and discovered that the 22 infants who had hMPV were poor inducers of inflammatory cytokines compared with the 46 infants who had RSV. The authors concluded that the viruses elicit disease by different mechanisms and therefore hMPV may augment RSV disease severity. To date, however, studies not only have not had the sample size to answer definitively if coinfection with hMPV and RSV increases bronchiolitis severity but also have been inadequate to determine the clinical implications of the many other pathogen combinations.

In a cooperative agreement with the National Institutes of Health, our research group, the Emergency Medicine Network (EMNet; www.emnet-usa.org), is currently conducting a prospective, multicenter study that will examine the clinical usefulness of testing for the causes of bronchiolitis in 2250 hospitalized children.[88] Based on the first year of our study, with a sample of 520 hospitalized children, we were able to detect a virus in 93% of the nasopharyngeal samples and found a 27% coinfection rate.[88] In the first year we have found that coinfection was significantly less likely for hospitalized children who had RSV (33%; 95% CI, 28%–38%) as compared with children who had RV (65%; 95%CI, 56%–73%).

WHEEZING AFTER SEVERE BRONCHIOLITIS

In 1959, Wittig and Glaser[89] noted a relationship between bronchiolitis and risk for asthma in 100 children in the United States. Over the past 50 years, several research groups have followed small cohorts of children hospitalized with bronchiolitis for the development of recurrent wheezing. For example, Carlsen and colleagues[90] found that 60% of 51 Norwegian infants hospitalized with bronchiolitis developed recurrent wheezing of childhood ($\geq$3 episodes of bronchial obstruction) by age 2 years compared with 4% of 24 control children. In a retrospective study from Qatar, 31 of 70 (44%) children younger than 12 months hospitalized with RSV bronchiolitis developed recurrent wheezing ($\geq$3 episodes of physician-diagnosed expiratory rhonchi) 2 years after admission, compared with 9 of the 70 controls (12%).[91] Sigurs and colleagues[92] followed a Swedish cohort of 47 infants hospitalized with RSV bronchiolitis and 93 controls up to age 13 years. At a mean age of 3 years, recurrent wheezing was diagnosed in 11 of 47 children (23%) in the RSV group versus 1 of 93 children (1%) in the control group.

Many of the children who have bronchiolitis who develop recurrent wheezing of childhood also develop childhood asthma. Unfortunately, the respiratory morbidity associated with childhood respiratory infections may be longstanding and influence the development and persistence of adult respiratory conditions.[93] In the Swedish cohort, the cumulative prevalence of asthma at age 7 years was 30% in the RSV group versus 3% in the control group[5] and at age 13 years the cumulative prevalence of asthma was 37% in the RSV group versus 5% among controls.[94] In the Tucson Children's Respiratory Study prospective birth cohort, having an RSV LRTI before age 3 years was an independent risk factor for wheezing up to age 11 years.[95] The association steadily subsides after age 3 years, however, and by age 13 years the association is no longer statistically significant.[95] Unlike the Swedish study, nearly all of the Tucson children who had RSV LRTI were not hospitalized and the respiratory utcomes of these two populations (ie, inpatient and outpatient) may be quite ifferent. Indeed, based on a Tennessee Medicaid database there is a dose–response elationship between bronchiolitis severity (as defined by inpatient, ED, and outpatient linic) and the increased odds of early childhood asthma and asthma-specific norbidity.[96]

Despite the generally strong associations, no one has been able to identify reliably he subset of children hospitalized with bronchiolitis at increased risk for developing ecurrent wheezing or if most of this large group of children will ultimately develop sthma.[97] Hampering this pursuit has been the terminology used to describe wheezing in preschool children[4] and the recent appreciation that asthma is a heterogeneous disease with multiple complex causes.[8,98,99]

HINOVIRUS BRONCHIOLITIS

lthough RSV is the most common pathogen associated with severe bronchiolitis[1,23] nd has been effectively used to define cohorts of children who have bronchioli- s,[28,91,92] other pathogens may have a stronger association with recurrent wheezing.[100–103] The most intriguing virus in studying recurrent wheezing and asthma RV. Several recent single-center studies have linked RV infection to asthma exacer- ations in children and adults,[104,105] infant wheezing,[68,106] and infants who have ecurrent respiratory symptoms and abnormal lung function.[107] Recent evidence so links LRTIs with RV-related wheezing in infancy to later development of recurrent wheezing of childhood[63] and asthma at age 6 years.[108–110] For example, in the Child- ood Origins of ASThma (COAST) birth cohort study, which involves 289 children at gh risk for developing asthma, the most significant independent predictor of recur- ent wheezing at age 3 years was a moderate to severe RV illness with wheezing uring infancy.[63] Furthermore, a Tennessee study showed that bronchiolitis during V-predominant months was associated with a 25% increased risk for childhood sthma over bronchiolitis during RSV-predominant months.[111] Our prospective multi- enter data of children younger than 2 years of age presenting to the ED with bron- niolitis found that children who have RV bronchiolitis have similar demographics, edical histories, and ED treatments as older children who have an asthma xacerbation.[67]

Of particular interest, and with potentially large clinical implications, are the results om one small trial of prednisolone for 3 days versus placebo for children hospitalized ith their first or second episode of wheezing due to RV. In this trial, Jartti, Lehtinen, id colleagues[112] found that children who had RV who received prednisolone had duced relapses during a 2-month period after the hospitalization and reduced recur- nt wheezing at 1 year.[113] Indeed, children who develop wheezing due to RV seem to ave a high likelihood of recurrent wheezing of childhood and eventually later devel- ping asthma.[110] Further investigation is warranted to clarify the potential value of tar- eting children who have RV bronchiolitis for the primary prevention of asthma.

Although this review focuses on viruses, we want to remind readers that the specific cteria colonizing an infant's hypopharynx also may play an important role in the risk r recurrent wheezing and childhood asthma.[114] In other words, a child's long-term utcome probably represents an interaction between the infecting virus, bacterial lieu (colonization or super-infection), and undoubtedly other factors (see Fig. 1).

TAMIN D AND WHEEZING

though there are many risk factors for the development of severe bronchiolitis[2,115] d the development of recurrent wheezing/asthma,[58,96,116–119] an emerging risk

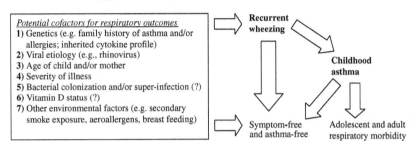

Severe Bronchiolitis

and

Potential cofactors for respiratory outcomes
1) Genetics (e.g. family history of asthma and/or allergies; inherited cytokine profile)
2) Viral etiology (e.g., rhinovirus)
3) Age of child and/or mother
4) Severity of illness
5) Bacterial colonization and/or super-infection (?)
6) Vitamin D status (?)
7) Other environmental factors (e.g. secondary smoke exposure, aeroallergens, breast feeding)

Recurrent wheezing

Childhood asthma

Symptom-free and asthma-free

Adolescent and adult respiratory morbidity

Fig. 1. Respiratory outcomes after severe bronchiolitis. After a child develops severe bronchiolitis (eg, an episode requiring hospitalization), several factors may influence the respiratory outcome. The actual percentages of children who develop each outcome remain unclear.

factor of particular interest to our research group is vitamin D status.[120] Vitamin D3 (cholecalciferol) comes from two sources: exposure to sunlight and dietary intake. The major source of vitamin D for most humans is from exposure of skin to the B fraction of ultraviolet light (UVB). In northern latitudes between November and March there are insufficient UVB rays to produce vitamin D, however.[121] Sunscreen use is recommended to protect against future skin cancer,[122–124] and this further decreases vitamin D skin production.[125] Unfortunately, lifestyle changes over the past few decades have made vitamin D deficiency increasingly common.[121,126,127]

The evidence for the possible link between vitamin D and respiratory disease comes from multiple studies. Two family-based studies demonstrated that gene polymorphisms on the vitamin D receptor were associated with childhood and adult asthma[128,129] and vitamin D deficiency is correlated with lower pulmonary function in adolescents[130] and adults.[131] Of greater relevance, Camargo and colleagues[132] discovered in a prospective birth cohort in Massachusetts that lower maternal intake of vitamin D during pregnancy is associated with increased risk for recurrent wheezing in the mothers' young children. These findings were replicated in 5-year-old Scottish children.[133] Camargo and colleagues[134] recently confirmed these novel findings in a separate birth cohort of 922 children from New Zealand (41°–43° S) where low 25-hydroxyvitamin D (25[OH]D) levels in cord blood were associated with increased risk for respiratory infections and childhood wheezing. Moreover, Litonjua and colleagues[135] recently examined the association between serum 25(OH)D levels and risk for an asthma-related ED visit or hospitalization. Among 1022 children who had asthma in the Childhood Asthma Management Program (CAMP),[136] those who had low baseline 25(OH)D levels (<75 nmol/L) were more likely to have a severe asthma exacerbation over a 4-month period (OR 1.50; 95%CI, 1.13–1.98). Finally, Brehm and colleagues[137] recently reported that among 616 children in Costa Rica who had asthma, higher 25(OH)D levels were significantly associated with reduced odds of any hospitalization and reduced use of anti-inflammatory medications.

The pathophysiology of these associations may relate to vitamin D's role in the activity of the innate immune system.[138–140] The innate immune system, specifically the activity of cathelicidin, helps prevent infections with bacteria and viruses.[141–145] In 2006, Liu and colleagues[146] reported in *Science* a link between Toll-like receptors (TLR), low vitamin D, and the reduced ability to support cathelicidin messenger RNA

duction. Wang and colleagues[138] also have demonstrated that vitamin D is a direct
ducer of the cathelicidin gene. Most recently, Janssen and colleagues determined
at single nucleotide polymorphisms in four of the innate immunity genes, including
e vitamin D receptor, helped predict susceptibility to RSV bronchiolitis.[147,148] Taken
gether, the clinical and mechanistic data support a role for vitamin D as an important
ctor in the relation between respiratory viruses in bronchiolitis and their link to recur-
ent wheezing.

SUMMARY

Bronchiolitis is the leading cause of hospitalization for children younger than 1 year of
ge and these hospitalized children have an increased risk for developing childhood
asthma. It remains unclear, however, which children who have severe bronchiolitis
eg, an episode requiring hospitalization) will develop recurrent wheezing or asthma.
Two intriguing factors are bronchiolitis due to RV and low levels of vitamin D. Devel-
ping a clearer understanding of the complex pathway from bronchiolitis to asthma
would help identify the subset of children who have severe bronchiolitis who are at
igh risk for developing asthma. This understanding would not only help clinicians
arget follow-up care but also advance bronchiolitis and asthma prevention research
by better routing high-risk children into future randomized trials.

REFERENCES

1. Glezen WP, Loda FA, Clyde WA Jr, et al. Epidemiologic patterns of acute lower
   respiratory disease of children in a pediatric group practice. J Pediatr 1971;
   78(3):397–406.
2. Carroll KN, Gebretsadik T, Griffin MR, et al. Increasing burden and risk factors for
   bronchiolitis-related medical visits in infants enrolled in a state health care insur-
   ance plan. Pediatrics 2008;122(1):58–64.
3. Singh AM, Moore PE, Gern JE, et al. Bronchiolitis to asthma: a review and call for
   studies of gene-virus interactions in asthma causation. Am J Respir Crit Care
   Med 2007;175(2):108–19.
4. Brand PL, Baraldi E, Bisgaard H, et al. Definition, assessment and treatment of
   wheezing disorders in preschool children: an evidence-based approach. Eur
   Respir J 2008;32(4):1096–110.
5. Sigurs N, Bjarnason R, Sigurbergsson F, et al. Respiratory syncytial virus bronchiolitis in infancy is an important risk factor for asthma and allergy at age 7.
   Am J Respir Crit Care Med 2000;161(5):1501–7.
6. Wainwright C, Isles AF, Francis PW. Asthma in children. Med J Aust 1997;167(4):
   218–23.
7. Yunginger JW, Reed CE, O'Connell EJ, et al. A community-based study of the
   epidemiology of asthma. Incidence rates, 1964–1983. Am Rev Respir Dis
   1992;146(4):888–94.
8. Martinez FD. Gene-environment interactions in asthma: with apologies to William
   of Ockham. Proc Am Thorac Soc 2007;4(1):26–31, PMCID: 2647610.
9. Yorita KL, Holman RC, Sejvar JJ, et al. Infectious disease hospitalizations among
   infants in the United States. Pediatrics 2008;121(2):244–52.
10. Diagnosis and management of bronchiolitis. Pediatrics 2006;118(4):1774–93.
11. Hanson IC, Shearer WT. Bronchiolitis. In: McMillan JA, DeAngelis CD, Feigin RD,
    et al, editors. Oski's pediatrics principles and practice. 3rd edition. Philadelphia:
    Lippincott Williams & Wilkins; 1999. p. 1214–6.

12. Fleisher GR. Infectious disease emergencies. In: Fleisher GR, Ludwig S, editors. Textbook of pediatric emergency medicine. 4th edition. Philadelphia: Lippincot Williams & Wilkins; 2000. p. 754–5.
13. Welliver R. Bronchiolitis and infectious asthma. In: Feigin R, Cherry J, Demmler G, et al, editors. Textbook of pediatric infectious diseases. 5th edition. Philadelphia: Saunders; 2004. p. 273–85.
14. Calogero C, Sly PD. Acute viral bronchiolitis: to treat or not to treat-that is the question. J Pediatr 2007;151(3):235–7.
15. Martinon-Torres F, Rodriguez-Nunez A, Martinon-Sanchez JM. Heliox therapy in infants with acute bronchiolitis. Pediatrics 2002;109(1):68–73.
16. Kuzik BA, Al-Qadhi SA, Kent S, et al. Nebulized hypertonic saline in the treatment of viral bronchiolitis in infants. J Pediatr 2007;151(3):266–70, 70 e1.
17. Corneli HM, Zorc JJ, Majahan P, et al. A multicenter, randomized, controlled trial of dexamethasone for bronchiolitis. N Engl J Med 2007;357(4):331–9.
18. Jartti T, Lehtinen P, Vuorinen T, et al. Bronchiolitis: age and previous wheezing episodes are linked to viral etiology and atopic characteristics. Pediatr Infect Dis J 2009;28(4):311–7.
19. Mansbach JM, Espinola JA, Macias CG, et al. Variability in the diagnostic labeling of nonbacterial lower respiratory tract infections: a multicenter study of children who presented to the Emergency Department. Pediatrics 2009;123:e573–81.
20. Shay DK, Holman RC, Newman RD, et al. Bronchiolitis-associated hospitalizations among US children, 1980–1996. JAMA 1999;282(15):1440–6.
21. Leader S, Kohlhase K. Respiratory syncytial virus-coded pediatric hospitalizations, 1997 to 1999. Pediatr Infect Dis J 2002;21(7):629–32.
22. Pelletier AJ, Mansbach JM, Camargo CA Jr. Direct medical costs of bronchiolitis hospitalizations in the United States. Pediatrics 2006;118(6):2418–23.
23. Hall CB, Walsh EE, Schnabel KC, et al. Occurrence of groups A and B of respiratory syncytial virus over 15 years: associated epidemiologic and clinical characteristics in hospitalized and ambulatory children. J Infect Dis 1990;162(6):1283–90.
24. Glezen WP, Taber LH, Frank AL, et al. Risk of primary infection and reinfection with respiratory syncytial virus. Am J Dis Child 1986;140(6):543–6.
25. Ukkonen P, Hovi T, von Bonsdorff CH, et al. Age-specific prevalence of complement-fixing antibodies to sixteen viral antigens: a computer analysis of 58,500 patients covering a period of eight years. J Med Virol 1984;13(2):131–48.
26. Levine DA, Platt SL, Dayan PS, et al. Risk of serious bacterial infection in young febrile infants with respiratory syncytial virus infections. Pediatrics 2004;113(6):1728–34.
27. Boyce TG, Mellen BG, Mitchel EF Jr, et al. Rates of hospitalization for respiratory syncytial virus infection among children in medicaid. J Pediatr 2000;137(6):865–70.
28. Wang EE, Law BJ, Stephens D. Pediatric Investigators Collaborative Network on Infections in Canada (PICNIC) prospective study of risk factors and outcomes in patients hospitalized with respiratory syncytial viral lower respiratory tract infection. J Pediatr 1995;126(2):212–9.
29. Willson DF, Horn SD, Hendley JO, et al. Effect of practice variation on resource utilization in infants hospitalized for viral lower respiratory illness. Pediatrics 2001;108(4):851–5.
30. Holman RC, Shay DK, Curns AT, et al. Risk factors for bronchiolitis-associated deaths among infants in the United States. Pediatr Infect Dis J 2003;22(6):483–90.

31. Shay DK, Holman RC, Roosevelt GE, et al. Bronchiolitis-associated mortality and estimates of respiratory syncytial virus-associated deaths among US children, 1979–1997. J Infect Dis 2001;183(1):16–22.
32. Papadopoulos NG, Bates PJ, Bardin PG, et al. Rhinoviruses infect the lower airways. J Infect Dis 2000;181(6):1875–84.
33. Korppi M, Kotaniemi-Syrjanen A, Waris M, et al. Rhinovirus-associated wheezing in infancy: comparison with respiratory syncytial virus bronchiolitis. Pediatr Infect Dis J 2004;23(11):995–9.
34. van den Hoogen BG, de Jong JC, Groen J, et al. A newly discovered human pneumovirus isolated from young children with respiratory tract disease. Nat Med 2001;7(6):719–24.
35. Thompson WW, Shay DK, Weintraub E, et al. Influenza-associated hospitalizations in the United States. JAMA 2004;292(11):1333–40.
36. Neuzil KM, Mellen BG, Wright PF, et al. The effect of influenza on hospitalizations, outpatient visits, and courses of antibiotics in children. N Engl J Med 2000;342(4):225–31.
37. Iwane MK, Edwards KM, Szilagyi PG, et al. Population-based surveillance for hospitalizations associated with respiratory syncytial virus, influenza virus, and parainfluenza viruses among young children. Pediatrics 2004;113(6):1758–64.
38. Rocholl C, Gerber K, Daly J, et al. Adenoviral infections in children: the impact of rapid diagnosis. Pediatrics 2004;113(1 Pt 1):e51–6.
39. Edwards KM, Thompson J, Paolini J, et al. Adenovirus infections in young children. Pediatrics 1985;76(3):420–4.
40. McIntosh K, Kapikian AZ, Turner HC, et al. Seroepidemiologic studies of coronavirus infection in adults and children. Am J Epidemiol 1970;91(6):585–92.
41. van der Hoek L, Pyrc K, Jebbink MF, et al. Identification of a new human coronavirus. Nat Med 2004;10(4):368–73.
42. Esper F, Weibel C, Ferguson D, et al. Evidence of a novel human coronavirus that is associated with respiratory tract disease in infants and young children. J Infect Dis 2005;191(4):492–8.
43. Woo PC, Lau SK, Chu CM, et al. Characterization and complete genome sequence of a novel coronavirus, coronavirus HKU1, from patients with pneumonia. J Virol 2005;79(2):884–95.
44. Lau SK, Woo PC, Yip CC, et al. Coronavirus HKU1 and other coronavirus infections in Hong Kong. J Clin Microbiol 2006;44(6):2063–71.
45. Esper F, Weibel C, Ferguson D, et al. Coronavirus HKU1 infection in the United States. Emerg Infect Dis 2006;12(5):775–9.
46. Allander T, Tammi MT, Eriksson M, et al. Cloning of a human parvovirus by molecular screening of respiratory tract samples. Proc Natl Acad Sci U S A 2005;102(36):12891–6.
47. Foulongne V, Rodiere M, Segondy M. Human bocavirus in children. Emerg Infect Dis 2006;12(5):862–3.
48. Bastien N, Brandt K, Dust K, et al. Human bocavirus infection, Canada. Emerg Infect Dis 2006;12(5):848–50.
49. Ma X, Endo R, Ishiguro N, et al. Detection of human bocavirus in Japanese children with lower respiratory tract infections. J Clin Microbiol 2006;44(3):1132–4.
50. Gaynor AM, Nissen MD, Whiley DM, et al. Identification of a novel polyomavirus from patients with acute respiratory tract infections. PLoS Pathog 2007;3(5):e64.
51. Allander T, Andreasson K, Gupta S, et al. Identification of a third human polyomavirus. J Virol 2007;81(8):4130–6, PMCID: 1866148.

52. Wattier RL, Vazquez M, Weibel C, et al. Role of human polyomaviruses in respiratory tract disease in young children. Emerg Infect Dis 2008;14(11):1766–8. PMCID: 2630739.
53. Duttweiler L, Nadal D, Frey B. Pulmonary and systemic bacterial co-infections in severe RSV bronchiolitis. Arch Dis Child 2004;89(12):1155–7, PMCID: 1719766.
54. Hall CB, Powell KR, Schnabel KC, et al. Risk of secondary bacterial infection in infants hospitalized with respiratory syncytial viral infection. J Pediatr 1988; 113(2):266–71.
55. Randolph AG, Reder L, Englund JA. Risk of bacterial infection in previously healthy respiratory syncytial virus-infected young children admitted to the intensive care unit. Pediatr Infect Dis J 2004;23(11):990–4.
56. Thorburn K, Harigopal S, Reddy V, et al. High incidence of pulmonary bacterial co-infection in children with severe respiratory syncytial virus (RSV) bronchiolitis. Thorax 2006;61(7):611–5.
57. Henrickson KJ, Hoover S, Kehl KS, et al. National disease burden of respiratory viruses detected in children by polymerase chain reaction. Pediatr Infect Dis J 2004;23(1 Suppl):S11–8.
58. Heymann PW, Carper HT, Murphy DD, et al. Viral infections in relation to age, atopy, and season of admission among children hospitalized for wheezing. J Allergy Clin Immunol 2004;114(2):239–47.
59. Jennings LC, Anderson TP, Werno AM, et al. Viral etiology of acute respiratory tract infections in children presenting to hospital: role of polymerase chain reaction and demonstration of multiple infections. Pediatr Infect Dis J 2004;23(11):1003–7.
60. Canducci F, Debiaggi M, Sampaolo M, et al. Two-year prospective study of single infections and co-infections by respiratory syncytial virus and viruses identified recently in infants with acute respiratory disease. J Med Virol 2008; 80(4):716–23.
61. Aberle JH, Aberle SW, Pracher E, et al. Single versus dual respiratory virus infections in hospitalized infants: impact on clinical course of disease and interferon-gamma response. Pediatr Infect Dis J 2005;24(7):605–10.
62. Williams JV, Harris PA, Tollefson SJ, et al. Human metapneumovirus and lower respiratory tract disease in otherwise healthy infants and children. N Engl J Med 2004;350(5):443–50.
63. Lemanske RF Jr, Jackson DJ, Gangnon RE, et al. Rhinovirus illnesses during infancy predict subsequent childhood wheezing. J Allergy Clin Immunol 2005; 116(3):571–7.
64. Legg JP, Warner JA, Johnston SL, et al. Frequency of detection of picornaviruses and seven other respiratory pathogens in infants. Pediatr Infect Dis J 2005;24(7):611–6.
65. Regamey N, Kaiser L, Roiha HL, et al. Viral etiology of acute respiratory infections with cough in infancy: a community-based birth cohort study. Pediatr Infect Dis J 2008;27(2):100–5.
66. Wolf DG, Greenberg D, Kalkstein D, et al. Comparison of human metapneumovirus, respiratory syncytial virus and influenza A virus lower respiratory tract infections in hospitalized young children. Pediatr Infect Dis J 2006;25(4):320–4.
67. Mansbach JM, McAdam AJ, Clark S, et al. Prospective multicenter study of the viral etiology of bronchiolitis in the emergency department. Acad Emerg Med 2008;15(2):111–8.
68. Kusel MM, de Klerk NH, Holt PG, et al. Role of respiratory viruses in acute upper and lower respiratory tract illness in the first year of life: a birth cohort study. Pediatr Infect Dis J 2006;25(8):680–6.

69. Jacobs JW, Peacock DB, Corner BD, et al. Respiratory syncytial and other viruses associated with respiratory disease in infants. Lancet 1971;1(7705):871–6.
70. Meissner HC, Murray SA, Kiernan MA, et al. A simultaneous outbreak of respiratory syncytial virus and parainfluenza virus type 3 in a newborn nursery. J Pediatr 1984;104(5):680–4.
71. Mufson MA, Krause HE, Mocega HE, et al. Viruses, Mycoplasma pneumoniae and bacteria associated with lower respiratory tract disease among infants. Am J Epidemiol 1970;91(2):192–202.
72. Ray CG, Minnich LL, Holberg CJ, et al. Respiratory syncytial virus-associated lower respiratory illnesses: possible influence of other agents. The Group Health Medical Associates. Pediatr Infect Dis J 1993;12(1):15–9.
73. Waner JL, Whitehurst NJ, Jonas S, et al. Isolation of viruses from specimens submitted for direct immunofluorescence test for respiratory syncytial virus. J Pediatr 1986;108(2):249–50.
74. Downham MA, Gardner PS, McQuillin J, et al. Role of respiratory viruses in childhood mortality. Br Med J 1975;1(5952):235–9.
75. Portnoy B, Eckert HL, Hanes B, et al. Multiple respiratory virus infections in hospitalized children. Am J Epidemiol 1965;82(3):262–72.
76. Subbarao EK, Griffis J, Waner JL. Detection of multiple viral agents in nasopharyngeal specimens yielding respiratory syncytial virus (RSV). An assessment of diagnostic strategy and clinical significance. Diagn Microbiol Infect Dis 1989;12(4):327–32.
77. Drews AL, Atmar RL, Glezen WP, et al. Dual respiratory virus infections. Clin Infect Dis 1997;25(6):1421–9.
78. Foulongne V, Guyon G, Rodiere M, et al. Human metapneumovirus infection in young children hospitalized with respiratory tract disease. Pediatr Infect Dis J 2006;25(4):354–9.
79. Greensill J, McNamara PS, Dove W, et al. Human metapneumovirus in severe respiratory syncytial virus bronchiolitis. Emerg Infect Dis 2003;9(3):372–5.
80. Semple MG, Cowell A, Dove W, et al. Dual infection of infants by human metapneumovirus and human respiratory syncytial virus is strongly associated with severe bronchiolitis. J Infect Dis 2005;191(3):382–6.
81. Poutanen SM, Low DE, Henry B, et al. Identification of severe acute respiratory syndrome in Canada. N Engl J Med 2003;348(20):1995–2005.
82. Guerrero-Plata A, Casola A, Garofalo RP. Human metapneumovirus induces a profile of lung cytokines distinct from that of respiratory syncytial virus. J Virol 2005;79(23):14992–7.
83. Alvarez R, Tripp RA. The immune response to human metapneumovirus is associated with aberrant immunity and impaired virus clearance in BALB/c mice. J Virol 2005;79(10):5971–8.
84. Douville RN, Bastien N, Li Y, et al. Human metapneumovirus elicits weak IFN-γ memory Responses compared with respiratory syncytial virus. J Immunol 2006;176(10):5848–55.
85. Mahalingam S, Schwarze J, Zaid A, et al. Perspective on the host response to human metapneumovirus infection: what can we learn from respiratory syncytial virus infections? Microbes Infect 2006;8(1):285–93.
86. Guerrero-Plata A, Casola A, Suarez G, et al. Differential response of dendritic cells to human metapneumovirus and respiratory syncytial virus. Am J Respir Cell Mol Biol 2006;34(3):320–9.
87. Laham FR, Israele V, Casellas JM, et al. Differential production of inflammatory cytokines in primary infection with human metapneumovirus and with other

common respiratory viruses of infancy. J Infect Dis 2004;189(11):2047–56 (Print).

88. Piedra P, Mansbach JM, Jewell A, et al. Prospective multicenter study of the etiology of bronchiolitis admissions 2007–2008. Baltimore (MD): Pediatric Academic Socieities; 2009.

89. Wittig HJ, Glaser J. The relationship between bronchiolitis and childhood asthma a follow-up study of 100 cases of bronchiolitis. J Allergy 1959;30(1):19–23.

90. Carlsen KH, Larsen S, Bjerve O, et al. Acute bronchiolitis: predisposing factors and characterization of infants at risk. Pediatr Pulmonol 1987;3(3):153–60.

91. Osundwa VM, Dawod ST, Ehlayel M. Recurrent wheezing in children with respiratory syncytial virus (RSV) bronchiolitis in Qatar. Eur J Pediatr 1993;152(12) 1001–3.

92. Sigurs N, Bjarnason R, Sigurbergsson F, et al. Asthma and immunoglobulin E antibodies after respiratory syncytial virus bronchiolitis: a prospective cohort study with matched controls. Pediatrics 1995;95(4):500–5.

93. Dharmage SC, Erbas B, Jarvis D, et al. Do childhood respiratory infections continue to influence adult respiratory morbidity? Eur Respir J 2009;33(2): 237–44.

94. Sigurs N, Gustafsson PM, Bjarnason R, et al. Severe respiratory syncytial virus bronchiolitis in infancy and asthma and allergy at age 13. Am J Respir Crit Care Med 2005;171(2):137–41.

95. Stein RT, Sherrill D, Morgan WJ, et al. Respiratory syncytial virus in early life and risk of wheeze and allergy by age 13 years. Lancet 1999;354(9178):541–5.

96. Carroll KN, Wu P, Gebretsadik T, et al. The severity-dependent relationship of infant bronchiolitis on the risk and morbidity of early childhood asthma. J Allergy Clin Immunol 2009;123(5):1055–61.

97. Frey U, Von Mutius E. The challenge of managing wheezing in infants. N Engl J Med 2009;360(20):2130–3.

98. Borish L, Culp JA. Asthma: a syndrome composed of heterogeneous diseases. Ann Allergy Asthma Immunol 2008;101(1):1–8 [quiz: 11, 50].

99. Reed CE. The natural history of asthma. J Allergy Clin Immunol 2006;118(3): 543–8 [quiz: 9–50].

100. Valkonen H, Waris M, Ruohola A, et al. Recurrent wheezing after respiratory syncytial virus or non-respiratory syncytial virus bronchiolitis in infancy: a 3-year follow-up. Allergy 2009 [epub ahead of print].

101. Reijonen TM, Korppi M. One-year follow-up of young children hospitalized for wheezing: the influence of early anti-inflammatory therapy and risk factors for subsequent wheezing and asthma. Pediatr Pulmonol 1998;26(2):113–9.

102. Reijonen TM, Kotaniemi-Syrjanen A, Korhonen K, et al. Predictors of asthma three years after hospital admission for wheezing in infancy. Pediatrics 2000; 106(6):1406–12.

103. Lee KK, Hegele RG, Manfreda J, et al. Relationship of early childhood viral exposures to respiratory symptoms, onset of possible asthma and atopy in high risk children: the Canadian asthma primary prevention study. Pediatr Pulmonol 2007;42(3):290–7.

104. Rawlinson WD, Waliuzzaman Z, Carter IW, et al. Asthma exacerbations in children associated with rhinovirus but not human metapneumovirus infection. J Infect Dis 2003;187(8):1314–8.

105. Venarske DL, Busse WW, Griffin MR, et al. The relationship of rhinovirus-associated asthma hospitalizations with inhaled corticosteroids and smoking. J Infect Dis 2006;193(11):1536–43.

06. Rakes GP, Arruda E, Ingram JM, et al. Rhinovirus and respiratory syncytial virus in wheezing children requiring emergency care. IgE and eosinophil analyses. Am J Respir Crit Care Med 1999;159(3):785–90.
07. Malmstrom K, Pitkaranta A, Carpen O, et al. Human rhinovirus in bronchial epithelium of infants with recurrent respiratory symptoms. J Allergy Clin Immunol 2006;118(3):591–6.
08. Roberg KA, Sullivan-Dillie KT, Evans MD, et al. Wheezing severe rhinovirus illnesses during infancy predict childhood asthma at age 6 years. J Allergy Clin Immunol 2007;119(1):619 [abstract].
09. Kotaniemi-Syrjanen A, Vainionpaa R, Reijonen TM, et al. Rhinovirus-induced wheezing in infancy—the first sign of childhood asthma? J Allergy Clin Immunol 2003;111(1):66–71.
10. Jackson DJ, Gangnon RE, Evans MD, et al. Wheezing rhinovirus illnesses in early life predict asthma development in high-risk children. Am J Respir Crit Care Med 2008;178(7):667–72.
111. Carroll KN, Wu P, Gebretsadik T, et al. Season of infant bronchiolitis and estimates of subsequent risk and burden of early childhood asthma. J Allergy Clin Immunol 2009;123(4):964–6.
112. Jartti T, Lehtinen P, Vanto T, et al. Evaluation of the efficacy of prednisolone in early wheezing induced by rhinovirus or respiratory syncytial virus. Pediatr Infect Dis J 2006;25(6):482–8.
113. Lehtinen P, Ruohola A, Vanto T, et al. Prednisolone reduces recurrent wheezing after a first wheezing episode associated with rhinovirus infection or eczema. J Allergy Clin Immunol 2007;119(3):570–5.
114. Bisgaard H, Hermansen MN, Buchvald F, et al. Childhood asthma after bacterial colonization of the airway in neonates. N Engl J Med 2007;357(15):1487–95.
115. Simoes EA. Environmental and demographic risk factors for respiratory syncytial virus lower respiratory tract disease. J Pediatr. 2003;143(5 Suppl):S118–26.
116. Martinez FD, Wright AL, Taussig LM, et al. Asthma and wheezing in the first six years of life. The Group Health Medical Associates. N Engl J Med 1995;332(3):133–8.
117. Guilbert TW, Morgan WJ, Zeiger RS, et al. Atopic characteristics of children with recurrent wheezing at high risk for the development of childhood asthma. J Allergy Clin Immunol 2004;114(6):1282–7.
118. Wu P, Dupont WD, Griffin MR, et al. Evidence of a causal role of winter virus infection during infancy in early childhood asthma. Am J Respir Crit Care Med 2008;178(11):1123–9.
119. Matricardi PM, Illi S, Gruber C, et al. Wheezing in childhood: incidence, longitudinal patterns and factors predicting persistence. Eur Respir J 2008;32(3):585–92.
120. Mansbach JM, Camargo CA Jr. Bronchiolitis: lingering questions about its definition and the potential role of vitamin D. Pediatrics 2008;122(1):177–9.
121. Webb AR, Kline L, Holick MF. Influence of season and latitude on the cutaneous synthesis of vitamin D3: exposure to winter sunlight in Boston and Edmonton will not promote vitamin D3 synthesis in human skin. J Clin Endocrinol Metab 1988;67(2):373–8.
122. Marks R, Jolley D, Lectsas S, et al. The role of childhood exposure to sunlight in the development of solar keratoses and non-melanocytic skin cancer. Med J Aust 1990;152(2):62–6.
123. Autier P, Dore JF. Influence of sun exposures during childhood and during adulthood on melanoma risk. EPIMEL and EORTC Melanoma Cooperative Group.

European Organisation for Research and Treatment of Cancer. Int J Cancer 1998;77(4):533–7.

124. Gilchrest BA, Eller MS, Geller AC, et al. The pathogenesis of melanoma induced by ultraviolet radiation. N Engl J Med 1999;340(17):1341–8.

125. Fuller KE, Casparian JM, Vitamin D. Balancing cutaneous and systemic considerations. South Med J 2001;94(1):58–64.

126. Lee JM, Smith JR, Philipp BL, et al. Vitamin D deficiency in a healthy group of mothers and newborn infants. Clin Pediatr (Phila) 2007;46(1):42–4.

127. Ziegler EE, Hollis BW, Nelson SE, et al. Vitamin D deficiency in breastfed infants in Iowa. Pediatrics 2006;118(2):603–10.

128. Poon AH, Laprise C, Lemire M, et al. Association of vitamin D receptor genetic variants with susceptibility to asthma and atopy. Am J Respir Crit Care Med 2004;170(9):967–73.

129. Raby BA, Lazarus R, Silverman EK, et al. Association of vitamin D receptor gene polymorphisms with childhood and adult asthma. Am J Respir Crit Care Med 2004;170(10):1057–65.

130. Burns J, Dockery D, Speizer FE. Low levels of dietary vitamin D intake and pulmonary function in adolescents. Proc Am Thorac Soc 2006;3:526 [abstract].

131. Black PN, Scragg R. Relationship between serum 25-hydroxyvitamin d and pulmonary function in the third national health and nutrition examination survey. Chest 2005;128(6):3792–8.

132. Camargo CA Jr, Rifas-Shiman SL, Litonjua AA, et al. Maternal intake of vitamin D during pregnancy and risk of recurrent wheeze in children at 3 y of age. Am J Clin Nutr 2007;85(3):788–95.

133. Devereux G, Litonjua AA, Turner SW, et al. Maternal vitamin D intake during pregnancy and early childhood wheezing. Am J Clin Nutr 2007;85(3):853–9.

134. Camargo CA Jr, Ingham T, Wickens K, et al. Cord blood 25-hydroxyvitamin D levels and risk of childhood wheeze in New Zealand. Am J Respir Crit Care Med. 2008;177(Suppl):A993 [abstract].

135. Litonjua AA, Hollis BW, Scheumann B, et al. Low serum vitamin D levels are associated with greater risks for severe exacerbations in childhood asthmatics. Am J Respir Crit Care Med 2008;177(suppl):A993 [abstract].

136. Long-term effects of budesonide or nedocromil in children with asthma. The Childhood Asthma Management Program Research Group. N Engl J Med 2000;343(15):1054–63.

137. Brehm JM, Celedon JC, Soto-Quiros ME, et al. Serum vitamin D levels and markers of severity of childhood asthma in Costa Rica. Am J Respir Crit Care Med 2009;179(9):765–71.

138. Wang TT, Nestel FP, Bourdeau V, et al. Cutting edge: 1,25-dihydroxyvitamin D3 is a direct inducer of antimicrobial peptide gene expression. J Immunol 2004; 173(5):2909–12.

139. Schauber J, Dorschner RA, Coda AB, et al. Injury enhances TLR2 function and antimicrobial peptide expression through a vitamin D-dependent mechanism. J Clin Invest 2007;117(3):803–11.

140. Martineau AR, Wilkinson KA, Newton SM, et al. IFN-γ- and TNF-independent vitamin D-inducible human suppression of Mycobacteria: the role of cathelicidin LL-37. J Immunol 2007;178(11):7190–8.

141. Ganz T. Defensins: antimicrobial peptides of innate immunity. Nat Rev Immunol 2003;3(9):710–20.

142. Nizet V, Ohtake T, Lauth X, et al. Innate antimicrobial peptide protects the skin from invasive bacterial infection. Nature 2001;414(6862):454–7.

43. Zhang L, Yu W, He T, et al. Contribution of human alpha-defensin 1, 2, and 3 to the anti-HIV-1 activity of CD8 antiviral factor. Science 2002;298(5595):995–1000.
44. Leikina E, Delanoe-Ayari H, Melikov K, et al. Carbohydrate-binding molecules inhibit viral fusion and entry by crosslinking membrane glycoproteins. Nat Immunol 2005;6(10):995–1001.
45. Bastian A, Schafer H. Human alpha-defensin 1 (HNP-1) inhibits adenoviral infection in vitro. Regul Pept 2001;101(1–3):157–61.
46. Liu PT, Stenger S, Li H, et al. Toll-like receptor triggering of a vitamin D-mediated human antimicrobial response. Science 2006;311(5768):1770–3.
47. Janssen R, Bont L, Siezen CL, et al. Genetic susceptibility to respiratory syncytial virus bronchiolitis is predominantly associated with innate immune genes. J Infect Dis 2007;196(6):826–34.
48. Roth DE, Jones AB, Prosser C, et al. Vitamin D receptor polymorphisms and the risk of acute lower respiratory tract infection in early childhood. J Infect Dis 2008;197:676–80.

ndex

Clin Lab Med 29 (2009) 757–765
doi:10.1016/S0272-2712(09)00108-5
0272-2712/09/$ – see front matter © 2009 Elsevier Inc. All rights reserved.

Moving?

Make sure your subscription moves with you!

To notify us of your new address, find your **Clinics Account Number** (located on your mailing label above your name), and contact customer service at:

Email: **journalscustomerservice-usa@elsevier.com**

800-654-2452 (subscribers in the U.S. & Canada)
314-447-8871 (subscribers outside of the U.S. & Canada)

Fax number: **314-447-8029**

Elsevier Health Sciences Division
Subscription Customer Service
3251 Riverport Lane
Maryland Heights, MO 63043

*To ensure uninterrupted delivery of your subscription, please notify us at least 4 weeks in advance of move.

Printed and bound by CPI Group (UK) Ltd, Croydon, CR0 4YY

08/06/2025

01896870-0013